IMMUNOLOGIC PROBLEMS

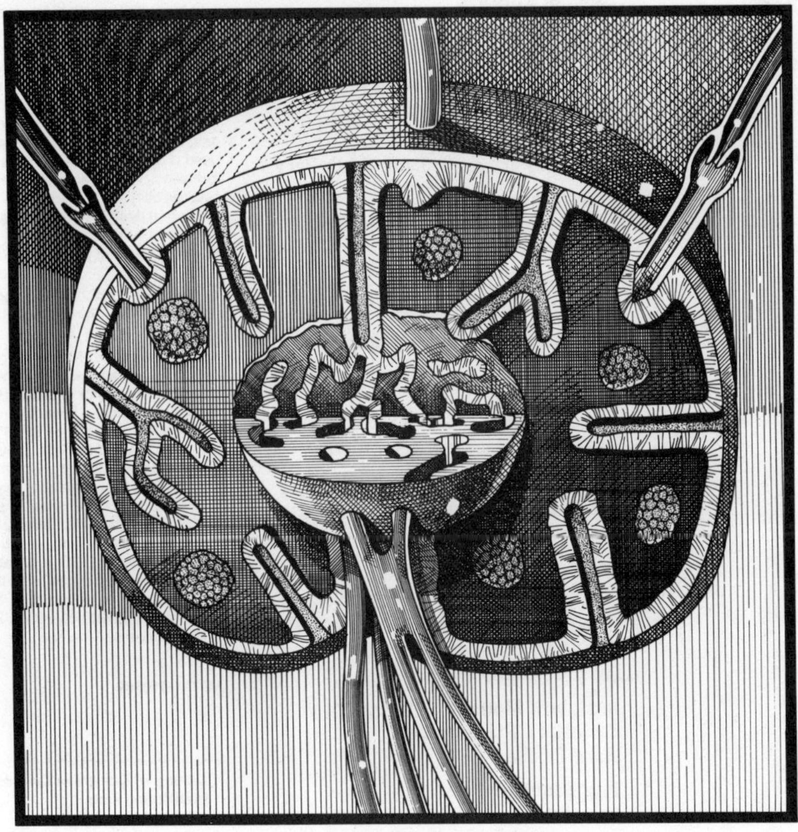

NurseReview™

Clinical Consultants for this section

John J. O'Shea, Jr., MD
Senior Staff Fellow, Cell Biology and Metabolism Branch, National Institutes of Health, Bethesda, Maryland

Paula Trahan Rieger, RN, OCN, BS, BSN, MSN
Clinical Nurse Specialist, Immunology and Chemopharmacology, M.D. Anderson Hospital and Tumor Institute, Houston, Texas

The clinical procedures described and recommended in this publication are based on research and consultation with medical and nursing authorities. To the best of our knowledge, these procedures reflect currently accepted clinical practice; nevertheless, they can't be considered absolute and universal recommendations. For individual application, treatment recommendations must be considered in light of the patient's clinical condition and, before administration of new or infrequently used drugs, in light of the latest package-insert information. The authors and the publisher disclaim responsibility for any adverse effects resulting directly or indirectly from the suggested procedures, from any undetected errors, or from the reader's misunderstanding of the text.

NRT11-010789

Library of Congress Cataloging-in-Publication Data
Immunologic problems.
p. cm.—(NurseReview)
Includes bibliographies and index.
1. Immunologic diseases 2. Immunologic diseases—Nursing. I. Springhouse Corporation. II. Series [DNLM: 1. Allergy and Immunology—nurses' instruction. QW504 I3316]
RC582.I468 1989 616.97 dc19
DNLM/DLC
ISBN 0-87434-220-1(SC) 88-20170

Contents

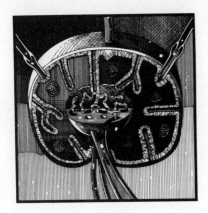

Fundamental Concepts

Autoimmune and Hypersensitivity Disorders

Immunodeficiency Disorders

Transplant- and Tumor-related Problems

Introduction

The immune system holds a pivotal position between health and illness. When working effectively, it continuously wards off disease and infection; when compromised, it leaves the body open to invasion from all types of pathogens. Understanding how the immune system works—and what can happen when it doesn't—will help you assess and care for patients with immunologic problems.

Written and reviewed by experts in the field, **Immunologic Problems** helps you understand the complexities of immune system function. It also helps bring you up to date on immunologic research, including the ongoing effort to understand and treat acquired immunodeficiency syndrome (AIDS). Throughout the book, you'll find information presented according to the nursing process, outlining your role every step of the way. Sample nursing care plans help you put nursing diagnoses into action by outlining patient goals, detailing nursing interventions, and specifying outcome criteria.

In the first chapter, you'll review the immune system's varied structures, including the thymus, bone marrow, lymph nodes, spleen, and mucosal-associated lymphoid tissue. You'll also review immune system cells, including lymphocytes, mononuclear phagocytes, polymorphonuclear granulocytes, and platelets. The chapter then goes on to explain specific immune responses, such as humoral and cell-mediated immunity, and nonspecific immune responses, such as inflammation and phagocytosis. In all, this review chapter will improve your understanding of the immune system and serves as a foundation for grasping concepts discussed in later chapters.

The next chapter, on autoimmunity, outlines what happens when the immune system produces antibodies against substances normally present in the body; the resulting tissue damage can range from minor local effects to potentially life-threatening systemic ones. The chapter offers many valuable pointers for accurate assessment, plus a discussion of pertinent diagnostic tests for autoimmune disorders. It then presents a comprehensive, nursing-oriented discussion of selected autoimmune disorders, starting with systemic lupus erythematosus. You'll find shorter discussions of rheumatoid arthritis, Sjögren's syndrome, Goodpasture's syndrome, and serum sickness. Descriptions and interventions for organ-specific autoimmune disorders appear in a convenient 5-page chart at the end of the chapter.

The following chapter addresses the four types of hypersensitivity reactions: immediate, cytotoxic, immune complex, and cell-mediated. A flow chart for each hypersensitivity type helps you understand just what happens in each one. You'll also find an in-depth discussion of anaphylaxis, including assessment, planning, intervention, and a sample care plan. You'll see how anaphylaxis develops and what systemic effects it produces. Other hypersensitivity disorders are covered in the chapter as well, including allergic rhinitis, urticaria, angioedema, hereditary angioedema, sarcoidosis, and hemolytic disease of the newborn.

Chapter 4 is devoted entirely to AIDS, the most challenging and controversial health care issue of our time. Here you'll learn the pathophysiology and epidemiology of human immunodeficiency vi-

Introduction

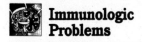

rus (HIV) infection, how the virus is transmitted, how it reproduces, and how it can lead to AIDS. You'll review the opportunistic infections commonly associated with AIDS. Most important, you'll learn to care for patients with AIDS—from assessment through interventions. The chapter also includes the Centers for Disease Control (CDC) definition of AIDS and CDC guidelines for protecting yourself from infection. Special sections deal with a potential HIV vaccine, patient teaching guidelines for condom use, and investigational AIDS drugs. The chapter ends with a discussion of pediatric AIDS and your role in caring for these children.

In chapter 5, the topic widens to primary and secondary immunodeficiency disorders: how to detect them and how to care for affected patients. Because immunosuppression heightens the risk of infection, the chapter presents several infection prevention and treatment measures. It then delves into the specifics of a score of primary immunodeficiency disorders. Secondary immunodeficiency disorders appear in a detailed chart at the end of the chapter.

The next chapter deals with immunologic problems of transplantation, particularly rejection. You'll find a discussion of the different types of rejection, including hyperacute, acute, and chronic. A full-page illustration uses kidney rejection to demonstrate the three rejection types. The text then explains how to assess and care for patients susceptible to rejection reactions. Another full-page illustration outlines signs and symptoms of rejection reactions throughout the body. Later in the chapter, you'll find a section devoted to recognizing and battling graft-versus-host disease, which can develop when an immunologically impaired patient receives an immunocompetent graft. Lastly, you'll find a chart that lists immunologic considerations for specific transplants, including bone and bone marrow, heart, kidney, liver, and pancreas.

In the book's final chapter, you'll discover how the immune system interacts with tumors. You'll review the antigenic properties of tumor cells, the immune response to tumor cells, and how the immune response helps in diagnosing and treating tumors. Special sections on tumor markers, interferon, interleukin-2, and monoclonal antibodies will build your understanding of tumor immunology.

Concluding with references and an index, **Immunologic Problems** promises to be an important and practical addition to your nursing library. Like all the other volumes in the NurseReview series, it provides a professional boost in today's challenging health care environment.

Immune System: An Overview

Geri Budesheim Neuberger and **JoAnn B. Reckling** wrote this chapter. An associate professor of medical-surgical nursing at the University of Kansas School of Nursing, Dr. Neuberger received her BA from Georgetown College (Ky.) and her MN and EdD from the University of Kansas. Ms. Reckling received her BSN from Ohio State University and her MN from the University of Kansas.

The body's bulwark against disease, the immune system guards against everything from cancer to the common cold. If we could unlock its secrets, we could perhaps cure some of our most dreaded diseases. But until that happens, no matter what your specialty, you'll be faced with unusual challenges and frustrations when caring for patients with immunologic problems. Even though we learn more about the immune system every day, we still know less about its interrelated workings than about any other body system.

To effectively care for patients with immune disorders, you'll first need to know how this complex system orchestrates the immune response. You'll find that information in this introductory chapter. Then, in later chapters, you'll find nursing information for specific immune disorders.

Defending against invasion

The immune system can't be separated into distinct compartments. Instead, it's a dynamic network with interrelated functions and actions. Immunity, in effect, includes all physiologic mechanisms that enable the body to recognize foreign substances and to neutralize, eliminate, or metabolize them. These mechanisms may cause injury to the body's own tissues—or they may not.

To accomplish its goals, the immune system must perform three main tasks:
- defense—resisting infection from microorganisms
- homeostasis—removing worn-out "self" components
- surveillance—recognizing and destroying mutant cells.

Normally, the skin and mucous membranes present an effective barrier against most foreign substances or microorganisms. However, if a foreign substance penetrates this barrier and enters the body, it triggers an immune response.

Immune system structures

The organs and cells involved in the immune response are referred to as the *lymphoid system*. These organs and cells exist as discrete capsules or simply as diffuse tissue accumulations. They're classified as primary and secondary lymphoid structures, depending on their function. (See *Classifying lymphoid structures*, page 4.)

Primary lymphoid structures

The site of lymphocyte and lymphatic tissue development, the primary lymphoid organs include the thymus and bone marrow.

Thymus. Located in the thorax overlying the heart and major vessels, the thymus consists of two pyramidal lobes encapsulated and partly divided by a thin layer of connective tissue. Peripheral portions of each lobule (cortex) are heavily infiltrated with lymphocytes; central portions (medulla) contain fewer lymphocytes. The medulla, though, is comparatively rich in hormone-producing epithelial cells. Also found in the thymus are keratin-containing cystic structures called Hassall's corpuscles, which also contribute to immune function.

Unlike other lymphoid organs, the thymus is shielded from contact with antigens and is composed of lymphoid and epithelial tissue.

Continued on page 5

Immunogenicity vs. antigenicity

Immunogenicity refers to an immunogen's ability to induce a specific immune response by producing antibodies, developing cell-mediated immunity, or both. Antigenicity refers to an antigen's ability to react with the products of a specific immune response (antibodies or sensitized T cells).

The two terms are often used interchangeably, but they shouldn't be. Although immunogenic substances are always antigenic, antigenic substances aren't always immunogenic. For instance, penicillin and other low-molecular-weight substances (haptens) aren't immunogenic unless attached to a larger carrier molecule. In such cases, haptens function as antigens but not as immunogens.

Immune System

Classifying lymphoid structures

Lymphoid structures can be classified as primary or secondary. Primary structures include the thymus and bone marrow, whereas secondary ones include the spleen, lymph nodes, and mucosal-associated lymphoid tissue (such as tonsils, adenoids, and Peyer's patches).

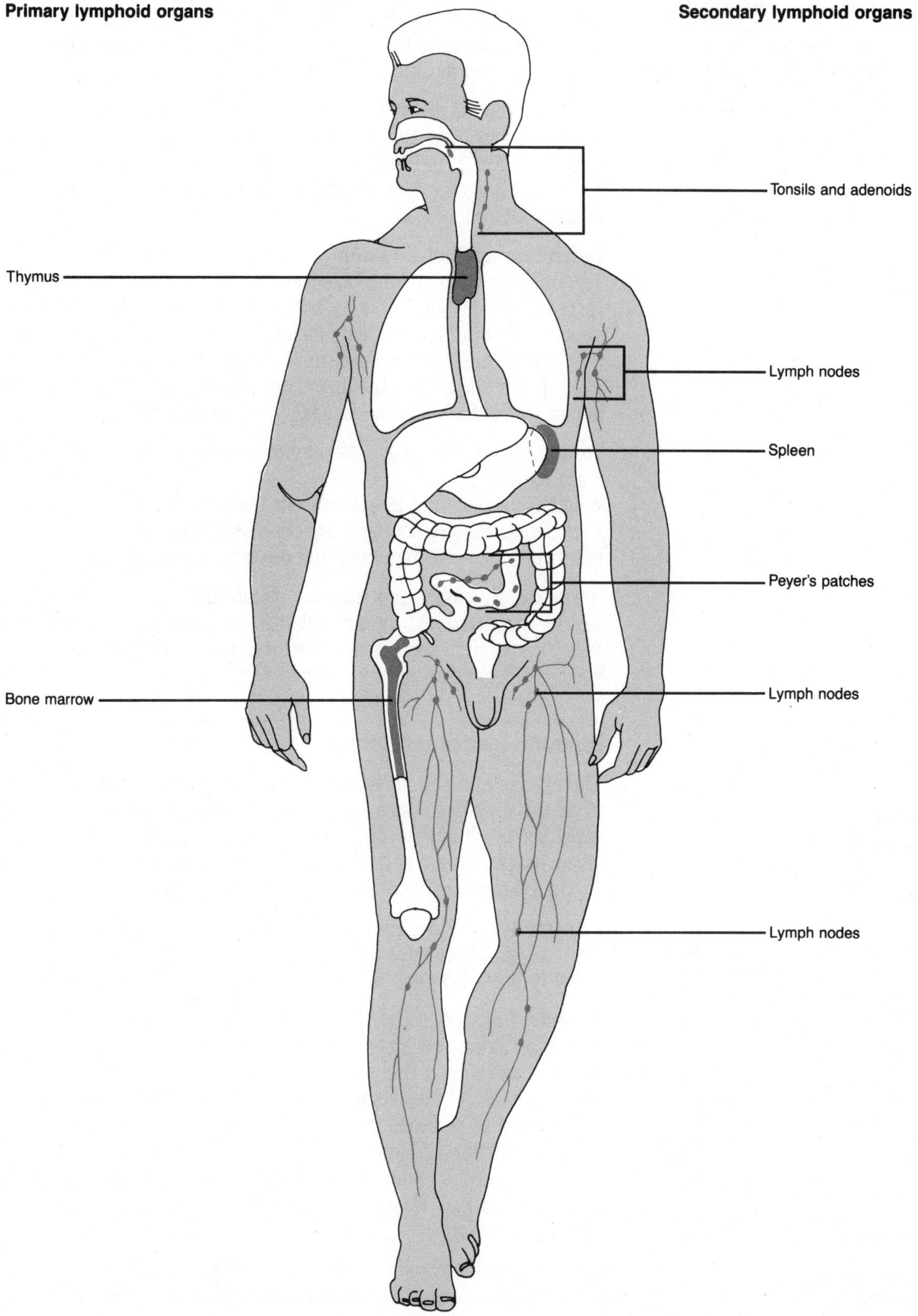

Immune System

Immune system structures—*continued*

Specifically, the thymus has two main functions:
- Its cortex produces T cells (T lymphocytes), which take part in the cell-mediated immune response. Even though T-cell precursors proliferate actively in the cortex, relatively small numbers reach the medulla to mature and subsequently enter the circulation.
- Its epithelial cells produce hormones, such as thymopoietin, thymic humoral factor, thymosin, and thymostimulin. These hormones affect T-cell differentiation.

The thymus also appears to direct immunogenesis in children and immune function in adults. It reaches full size at puberty and progressively decreases thereafter. This parallels the reduction in lymphoid tissue and antibodies that accompanies aging.

Bone marrow. Soft organic material, marrow fills bone cavities throughout the body and produces precursors of lymphocytes (called stem cells). Bone marrow is involved in antigen processing, cell-mediated and humoral immunity, and recognition and removal of worn-out cells.

Secondary lymphoid structures

Secondary structures include the lymph nodes, spleen, and mucosal-associated tissue, such as the tonsils and Peyer's patches in the intestine. These organs and tissues promote lymphocytic interactions as well as lymphocyte-antigen interactions. They also disseminate the immune response once it's generated.

Lymph nodes. Distributed throughout the body, lymph nodes are oval structures through which lymphocytes pass. The lymph node consists of an outer portion (cortex) and an inner portion (medulla), which are surrounded by a connective tissue capsule with protruding trabeculae. The capsule provides support and creates a conduit for blood vessels. After exposure to antigens, nodules develop along the lymph node's periphery. These nodules are composed of large numbers of lymphocytes.

In the nodule's center are collections of actively dividing cells called germinal centers. These centers contain B cells and, along with the deeper medullary region, are called the *bursal equivalent tissues*. Deeper cortical zones, known as paracortical or subcortical regions, contain venules, through which the lymphocytes pass from the blood lymph. Called the thymic-dependent region, these areas contain T cells.

The lymph node has two main functions:
- filtration of foreign material
- circulation of lymphocytes.

Lymphocytes enter the lymph node through the vascular system and the lymphatics. They progressively enrich the lymph circulating through the lymphatics. When this lymphocyte-enriched lymph empties into the bloodstream from the thoracic ducts, it's quite different from its origin as tissue fluid. Lymphocytes are also added from the venules, becoming part of a recirculating lymphocyte pool that

Continued on page 6

Immune System

Immune system structures—*continued*

travels from the blood to the lymph and then back to the blood. This recirculating lymphocyte pool primarily consists of T cells.

Spleen. The only blood-filtering lymphatic organ, the spleen lies in the left upper abdominal quadrant, behind the stomach and near the diaphragm. Trabeculae encapsulate the organ and extend inward. Arterial blood travels along the trabeculae after entering the spleen through the hilus.

Like the lymph nodes, the spleen produces lymphocytes and plasma cells. Besides its phagocytic function, the spleen responds to antigenic stimulation and also performs such nonimmune functions as removing worn-out cells from the blood, converting hemoglobin to bilirubin, and releasing iron into the blood for reuse.

The spleen's interior or pulp is filled with two kinds of tissue: white and red. White pulp serves as the spleen's main site for lymphocyte deposition. Bursal equivalent tissues are found in the white pulp and contain B cells; other lymphocytes, surrounding the follicles and periarteriolar sheaths, contain T cells and are referred to as the thymic-dependent regions. The white pulp also includes lymph nodules. Sheaths of white pulp and lymphocytes surround the smaller splenic arteries, which branch off into capillaries and enter the lymph nodules.

Red pulp, which surrounds white pulp, contains large numbers of erythrocytes and helps to filter them from the blood. As blood courses through the red pulp, it accumulates components responsible for phagocytosis.

Mucosal-associated lymphoid tissue (MALT). Typically, mucosal surfaces offer easy access for invading microbes and other foreign substances. To combat these antigens, MALT carries out a local immune response. MALT consists mainly of diffuse aggregates of nonencapsulated lymphoid tissue but, in a few areas, it forms nodules with germinal centers. This lymphoid tissue appears most commonly in these submucosal areas:

- the GI tract, as gut-associated lymphoid tissue (GALT). GALT occurs throughout the intestine in multiple lymphoid aggregates, such as Peyer's patches, or in nodules, such as the isolated lymphoid follicles found mainly in the colon. It promotes production of secretory immunoglobulin A (IgA) and helps develop tolerance to ingested antigens.
- the bronchi, as bronchus-associated lymphoid tissue (BALT). BALT appears in the lower respiratory tract and hilar lymph nodes. It's associated mainly with IgA production in response to inhaled antigens.
- the skin, as skin-associated lymphoid tissue (SALT). Antigens that enter the body through epidermal Langerhans' cells interact with lymphocytes in the skin and with draining lymph nodes.

Smaller amounts of MALT appear at other vulnerable sites, such as the middle ear, mammary glands, conjunctiva, salivary glands, and parts of the urogenital tract.

Immune System

Lymphoid system cells

Derived from pluripotential (undifferentiated) stem cells, the cells involved in the lymphoid system and immune response include lymphocytes, mononuclear phagocytes, polymorphonuclear granulocytes, and platelets. (See *How lymphoid cells develop*, page 8.)

Lymphocytes

Lymphocytes develop in the primary lymphoid organs, T cells in the thymus, and B cells in the bursa of fabricus or bursal equivalent in mammals. They then migrate to the secondary tissues where they can respond to antigen. Lymphocytes associated with the immune response include T cells, B cells, null cells, and T-cell and B-cell products called lymphokines.

T cells. These cells have effector and regulatory functions. Effector functions result from T-cell ability to secrete proteins (lymphokines) and to kill other cells (cytotoxic function). These functions include reactivity, such as delayed hypersensitivity reactions, allograft rejections, tumor immunity, and graft-versus-host reactions. In their regulatory function, T cells can boost the cytotoxicity of other T cells and B-cell production of immunoglobulin. These functions also require lymphokine synthesis.

Most T cells spend much of their lives in the thymus, where they differentiate into mature cells. Stem cells called thymocytes travel to the thymus from the bone marrow, then from the cortex to the medulla, and then into the bloodstream over about 3 days. The vast majority of these cells quickly die; about 10% enter the bloodstream as mature, functional T cells with developed antigen receptors and, thus, the ability to respond to specific antigens. These mature T cells enter the bloodstream through the walls of the medulla's venules. From the bloodstream, T cells disperse into the peripheral lymphoid tissues, gathering in the inner cortex of the lymph nodes, periarterial sheaths of the spleen, or intranodular areas of Peyer's patches. However, in less than 24 hours, T cells begin their return journey to the bloodstream. They leave the lymphoid tissues by way of efferent lymphatics and then travel to the larger lymphatics, the thoracic duct, and on to the bloodstream.

During T-cell development in the thymic cortex, CD molecules (formerly called T molecules) appear on the T-cell surface. CD2 (T11) molecules appear first, followed by CD3 (T3), CD4 (T4), and CD8 (T8). Other accessory molecules, including CD25 and Ti, may also appear. When the T cell reaches the medulla, it follows one of two even more specialized developmental paths, becoming a $CD4^+$ and $CD8^-$ or $CD4^-$ and $CD8^+$ variant. Both variants carry CD2 and CD3 molecules.

What's the significance of these CD lineages? The significance lies in the T cells' eventual roles. Cells of the $CD2^+$, $CD3^+$, $CD4^+$ variety, which make up 65% of circulating T cells, act as T-helper (or T-inducer) cells, promoting antibody production. Cells of the $CD2^+$, $CD3^+$, $CD8^+$ variety, which make up about 35% of circulating T cells, function as T-suppressor or T-cytotoxic cells, suppressing antibody production or destroying target cells.

Continued on page 9

Immune System

How lymphoid cells develop

From a pluripotential stem cell come two main cell systems: hematopoietic and lymphopoietic. The hematopoietic system produces cells responsible for inflammation and phagocytosis. The lymphopoietic system produces cells responsible for humoral and cell-mediated immunity.

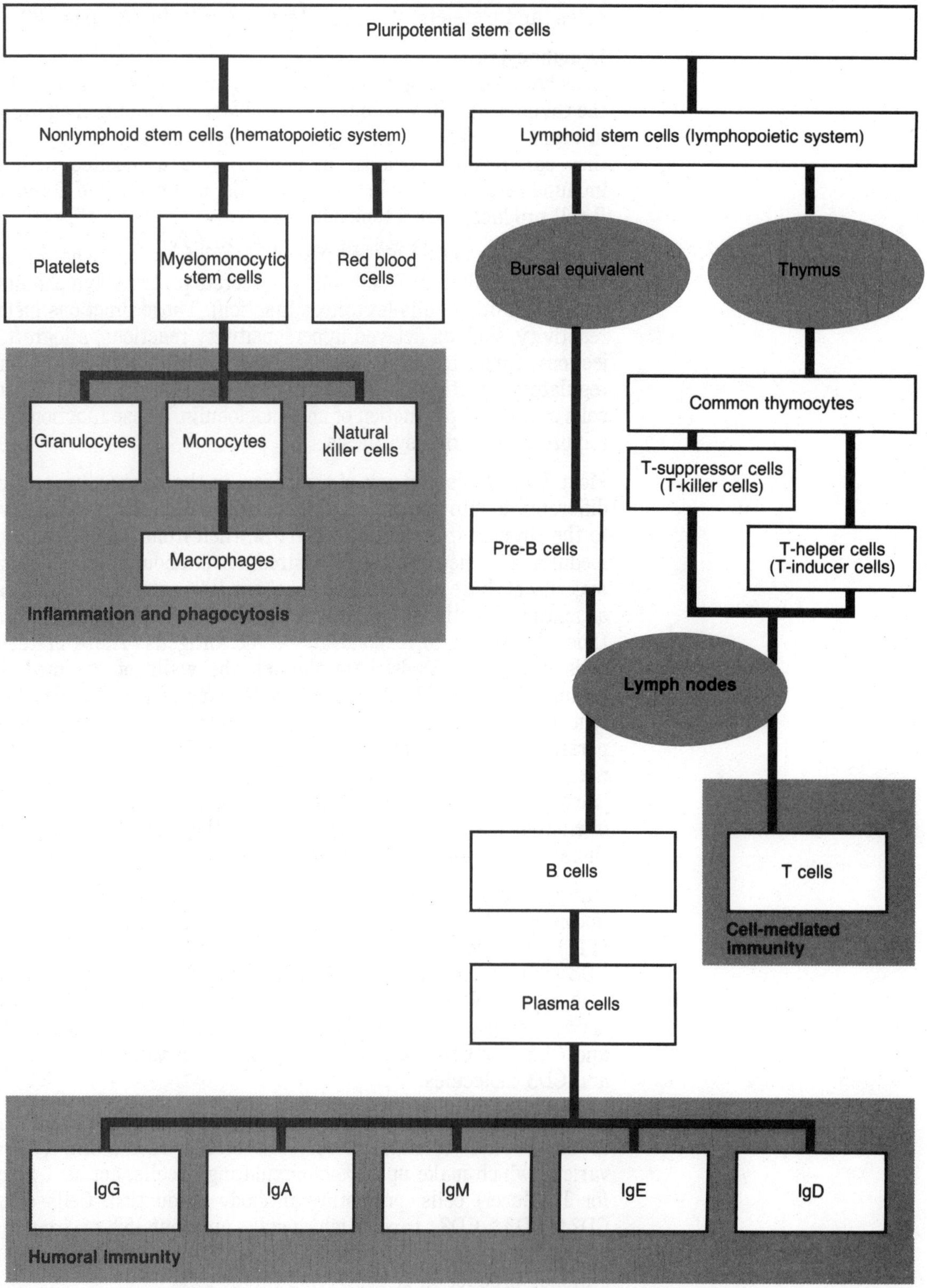

Immune System

Major histocompatibility complex

The major histocompatibility complex (MHC), located on the short arm of chromosome 6, consists of genes that code for the cell surface expression of strong transplantation antigens as well as histocompatibility-linked immune response genes. In effect, the MHC controls antigen synthesis and graft rejection in transplants. It also affects the immune response to infections and susceptibility to immunologically mediated diseases. In man, the MHC system is called the *human leukocyte antigen (HLA) system.*

MHC genes code for three classes of antigens:

Class I antigens, also called the classic histocompatibility antigens, include the HLA-A, HLA-B, and HLA-C antigens. Located on nucleated cells, these antigens are the principal ones identified by the host during graft rejection. They're also the antigens targeted by killer T cells. These antigens help the immune system recognize and eliminate virally infected cells.

Class II antigens, also called Ia antigens, include the HLA-D, HLA-DR, HLA-DQ, and HLA-DP antigens. They're mainly located on the outside of immunocompetent cells, including macrophages, monocytes, resting T cells, activated T cells, and especially B cells. They probably influence the sensitization phase of cell-mediated cytolysis; they play a part in antigen presentation by macrophages to T cells; and they foster collaboration between immunocompetent cells. However, the HLA-DP antigens differ from all others in Class II because they can evoke a strong secondary proliferative response and act as targets for killer T cells.

Class III antigens include the second and fourth components (C2 and C4) of the classic complement pathway and the properdin factor B of the alternative pathway. (For more details on Class III antigens, see the section on complement in this chapter.)

Lymphoid system cells—*continued*

T cells recognize specific antigens by means of a receptor called the α/β heterodimer, which is located at the end of each CD molecule. However, this receptor doesn't recognize antigen alone. Instead, it recognizes antigen along with the products of major histocompatibility complex (MHC) genes. For viral antigens, recognition occurs in conjunction with Class I MHC molecules; for soluble antigen, in conjunction with Class II MHC molecules. Large soluble antigens may also need processing by a macrophage, branched (dendritic) cell, or other accessory cell.

First, an antigen must undergo phagocytosis by an antigen-presenting cell, which engulfs, processes, and expresses the antigen on its own cell surface together with Class I or II MHC molecules. (See *Major histocompatibility complex.*) After phagocytosis, the α/β heterodimer can then recognize the antigen along with the "self" MHC molecules. CD4 molecules recognize Class II MHC molecules; CD8 molecules recognize Class I MHC molecules. What's more, CD4 molecules help B cells develop into immunoglobulin-secreting (antibody-secreting) plasma cells, whereas CD8 molecules suppress this differentiation. The CD2 molecules' role isn't clear. CD3 molecules may help in recognizing antigens or MHC molecules and in stabilizing the antigen receptor.

B cells. Derived from bone marrow or bursa equivalent, B cells function as specific antigen receptors using endogenous immunoglobulins that evolve on their surface membranes. B cells are thymic-independent immunoglobulin-producing cells. (See *Immunoglobulin structure*, page 10, and *Antibody variants*, page 11.)

B cells begin to form before birth, generated from the fetal liver after hematopoietic stem cells travel there from the yolk sac. In fact, the fetal liver produces the majority of red blood (erythroid) cells, bone marrow (myeloid) cells, and B cells until well into the second trimester of gestation. Thereafter, bone marrow produces B cells and other types of blood cells, continuing this function throughout life. B cells arise from the same pluripotential stem cells that produce other hematopoietic and lymphopoietic cells, developing from precursor B (pre-B) to immature, to mature, and to activated B cells.

After antigenic stimulation, B cells either differentiate into plasma cells, which excrete large amounts of immunoglobulin, or divide and return to a resting state as small, postmitotic B cells called memory B cells. Upon second exposure to the same antigen, memory B cells can quickly differentiate into plasma cells. This accounts for the more rapid, intense antibody response that occurs after this second exposure.

Plasma cells rarely divide, so they usually live less than 4 days. Most mature plasma cells reside in such lymphoid tissues as the medullary cords of the lymph nodes, the red pulp areas of the spleen, the lamina propria of the intestinal and respiratory tracts, and the bone marrow sinusoids. Few appear in the circulation.

B-cell activation involves a number of stimulating factors. Although B cells do develop without antigenic or environmental stimulation,

Continued on page 10

Immune System

Immunoglobulin structure

Glycoproteins that combine with antigens, immunoglobulins consist of 82% to 96% polypeptide and 4% to 18% carbohydrate. One part of the immunoglobulin molecule (the antigen-binding site) controls binding to antigen; the other part controls binding to host tissues, including immune system cells, phagocytic cells, and the first component (C1q) of the classic complement pathway. Antigen specificity is governed by the amino acid sequence at the antigen-binding site.

All immunoglobulin molecules consist of two identical light polypeptide chains and two identical heavy polypeptide chains connected by disulfide bonds. The molecules are mainly divided into classes and subclasses according to the type of heavy polypeptide chain. Five types of heavy chains and two types of light chains exist. These chains are divided into a constant region (C) and a variable region (V), with antigen-binding sites located on the variable region.

The enzyme papain separates the IgG molecule's heavy chain into two parts at the hinge region, creating one Fc (crystallizable) fragment and two Fab (antigen-binding) fragments. The enzyme pepsin further separates the molecule, creating an Fab′ 2 fragment.

Five different classes of immunoglobulins exist: IgG, IgA, IgM, IgD, and IgE. These classes differ in size, charge, amino acid composition, and carbohydrate content. IgG, IgD, and IgE have two antigen-binding sites per molecule, IgM has ten sites per molecule, and dimeric class IgA (usually found in secretions) has four combining sites per molecule. IgG, IgD, and IgE exist only as monomers of the four-chain unit; IgM exists as a pentamer with five connected four-chain units; and IgA exists in both monomeric and polymeric forms.

Basic immunoglobulin structure (IgG, IgD, IgE)

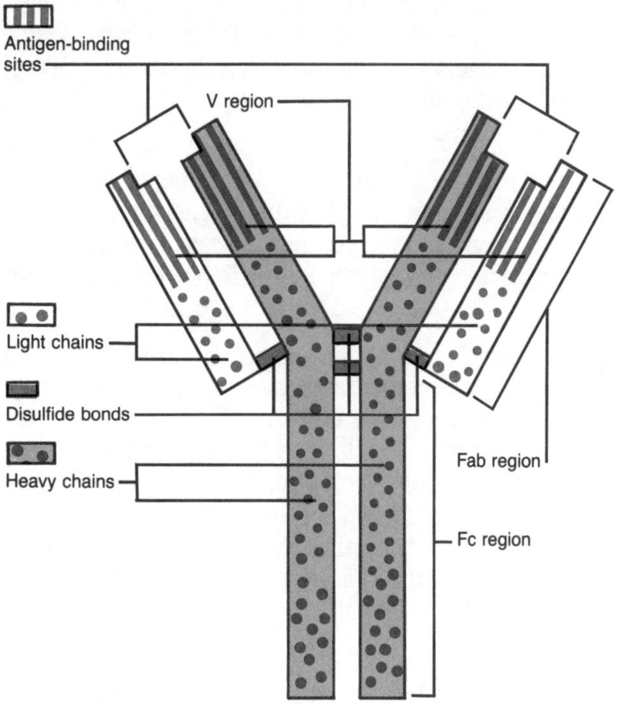

IgM structure

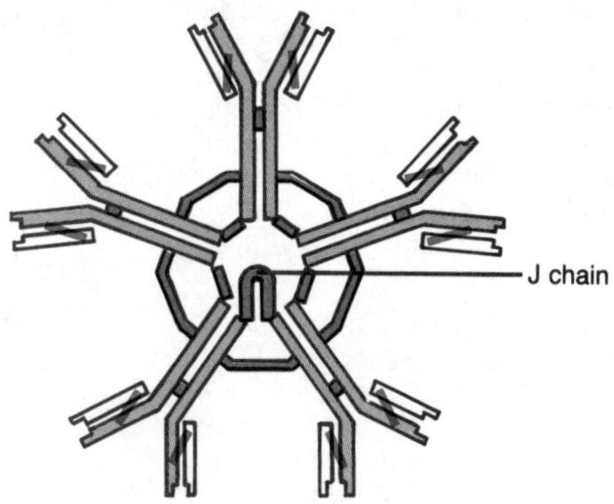

IgA structure

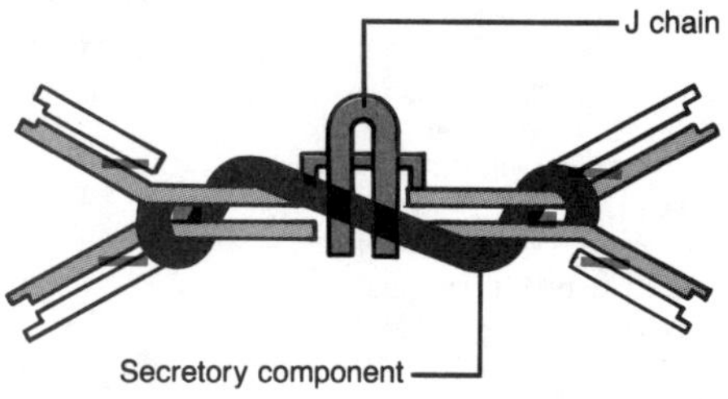

Lymphoid system cells—*continued*

antigens and other mitogens play a fundamental role in spurring resting B cells to proliferate and differentiate further.

Once a B cell is activated, a series of changes takes place on its surface that controls the progression of the cell's response. Electrical depolarization of the membrane, one of the first changes, is followed a few hours later by a sharp increase in the surface density of Class II MHC molecules, essential for B-cell and T-cell interaction. Later, B cells acquire surface receptors for growth and differentiation-promoting factors produced by activated T cells; these factors include transferrin, interleukin-2, and others. Other apparently crucial molecules for B-cell activation include interleukin-1 and gamma-

Immune System

Antibody variants

Antibody variants come in three types: isotypic, allotypic, and idiotypic.

Isotypic variations refer to the differences in heavy and light chain classes and subclasses. Genes for these variants exist in all healthy members of a species.

Also called genetic markers, *allotypic (allelic) variations* refer to the genetic differences between alleles of a species at a given locus. Not all healthy members of a species have genes for these variations; for instance, allotypic forms are found in blood groups. They've been found on both the heavy and light chains of the IgG and IgA molecules. Factors associated with the heavy chain of IgG are called Gm; those associated with the light chain are called Inv. More than 20 Gm factors and 3 Inv factors exist. The factors associated with the IgA molecule are called Am.

Idiotypic variations denote the unique V-region sequences created by each clone of antibody-forming cells. They're probably associated with the hypervariable regions that determine antibody specificity.

interferon, which we'll discuss shortly. What's more, recent evidence shows that activated B cells generate some of their own growth factors, and that glucocorticoids can encourage activated B cells to differentiate into plasma cells.

T cells also help antigen-induced B-cell responses. These responses include an outpouring of signals started when soluble ligands (molecules that react to form a complex with another molecule) bind to B-cell receptors. After antigens bind to B-cell surface antibodies, they're internalized, partly degraded, and recycled in fragments to the B-cell surface along with Class II MHC molecules. The T cell's antigen receptor can then recognize a combination of Class II MHC molecules and processed antigen.

Bonds formed between CD4 molecules on T-helper cells and a specialized area on the Class II MHC molecules of B cells may help stabilize the interaction between T cells and B cells. Activated T-helper cells generate soluble factors that bind to specific receptors on activated B cells, prompting them to grow and differentiate.

T cells promote immunoglobulin production by directly interacting with B cells and by secreting soluble regulatory materials. In fact, direct contact between antigen-specific T cells and antigen-specific B cells may be necessary to start B-cell activation. This initial activation results in expression of certain receptors on the B-cell surface that bind to growth and differentiation factors released by T cells. These factors cause specific B-cell clones to multiply and expand and encourage B cells to differentiate into immunoglobulin-secreting plasma cells.

Immunoglobulins. The five classes of immunoglobulins include IgG, IgA, IgM, IgD, and IgE. These classes differ in size, charge, amino acid composition, and carbohydrate content.

IgG, the main serum immunoglobulin, makes up 70% to 75% of the total immunoglobulin pool and has four subclasses (IgG_1, IgG_2, IgG_3, IgG_4). High concentrations appear in both vascular and extravascular spaces. IgG has a relatively long half-life of 23 days, crosses the placenta (protecting newborns during the first 3 to 6 months of life), and activates complement by functioning as an opsonin. It's believed to build up immunity against bacteria, viruses, parasites, fungi, and other blood-borne infecting agents. It also causes antibody activity in tissues. IgG receptors are found on monocytes, polymorphonuclear leukocytes, reticuloendothelial cells in the liver and spleen, and some lymphocytes.

IgA, the second most plentiful serum immunoglobulin, accounts for 15% to 20% of the total immunoglobulin pool and has two subclasses (IgA_1, IgA_2). It's produced by the lymphoid tissues lining the GI, respiratory, and genitourinary tracts. Its most important contribution to immunity is in the external secretory system. IgA mixes with a protein called secretory component or secretory IgA (sIgA) in saliva, tears, bronchial and vaginal secretions, nasal mucosa, and prostatic fluid to ease its transport into secretions and to protect it against the proteolytic enzymes usually found in these areas. IgA molecules activate complement by the alternate pathway. They don't cross the placenta, but they do enhance the immunity

Continued on page 12

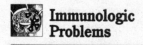

Immune System

Lymphoid system cells—*continued*

of newborns because of their high colostrum levels. IgA receptors appear on lymphocytes, polymorphonuclear leukocytes, and monocytes.

IgM, the largest immunoglobulin, makes up about 10% of the immunoglobulin pool. Its size limits it almost completely to the intravascular space. IgM molecules are extremely effective agglutinators of particulate immunogens, such as bacteria and red blood cells; they also efficiently fix complement. However, unlike IgG molecules, they aren't opsonins. The surface receptor for B cells, IgM is synthesized before IgG in early primary immune responses to most antigens, and is also important in certain antibody responses such as "natural" blood group antibodies.

Although IgD makes up less than 1% of total immunoglobulin, it's nonetheless found in large quantities on many circulating B-cell membranes. Its exact function isn't known, but this immunoglobulin may be important in antigen-provoked lymphocyte differentiation. IgD appears on the surface of B cells, particularly in neonates. It has two subclasses (IgD_1, IgD_2).

Found only in trace amounts in serum, IgE is associated with immediate hypersensitivity reactions. It's primarily produced in the respiratory and intestinal tract linings and is part of the external antibody secretory system. It binds to high-affinity receptors and is located on the surface membranes of basophils and mast cells.

Null cells. Also called non-T, non-B cells or third-population cells, null cells differ from both T cells and B cells. Null cells are hematopoietic stem cells, and may include T-cell and B-cell precursors, myeloid cells, erythroid cells, and platelet (thrombocytic) cells. Null cells can destroy tumor cells either spontaneously or through an antibody-dependent cellular cytotoxic (ADCC) mechanism. These cells come in two types: killer (K) cells and natural killer (NK) cells.

K cells. Although K cell origin is unknown, these cells are known to be cytotoxic to target cells coated with IgG in an ADCC reaction. In this reaction, an antibody molecule appears to form a bridge between the target cell and the effector cell.

NK cells. Like K cells, NK cells have an unknown origin. These cells have no known T-cell or B-cell markers and don't need to be sensitized before generation. They may be involved in nonspecific killing of virally transformed target cells, in allograft and tumor rejection, and in resistance to some infections. They also may prove important in immune surveillance of malignant diseases.

Lymphokines. Produced throughout the body, lymphokines exert both local and systemic effects. Also called cytokines, these nonspecific, soluble mediators function as intracellular signals that regulate local and, at times, systemic inflammatory responses. They influence immunity and inflammation by directing the growth, movement, and differentiation of leukocytes and nonleukocytic cells.

Monoclonal antibody

A homogenous antibody to a specific antigen, a monoclonal antibody has its origin in a hybridoma, created when a normal antibody-secreting B cell fuses with an animal or human myeloma cell. The resulting product has the antigenic specificity of antibody secreted by B cells.

As the name *monoclonal* suggests, the homogeneous immunoglobulin results from multiplication of a single plasma-cell clone. The proteins produced can be complete immunoglobulin molecules, free light chains (Bence Jones proteins), or both. In rare conditions, such as heavy-chain disease, only parts of immunoglobulin chains are formed.

Researchers have made the following observations about monoclonal antibodies:
- They seem to be normal immunoglobulins. Although they're different from pools of immunoglobulin, they don't display an unusual pathology.
- Many have antibody activity.

One of the most exciting recent advances in immunology has been the discovery of a way to produce large amounts of monoclonal antibody in vitro. Today, these antibodies are being used extensively as diagnostic and therapeutic reagents. For example, they're used as serologic reagents to identify infectious agents, tumor antigens, histocompatibility antigens, and functional subpopulations of lymphoid cells. They're also used to help treat lymphomas, acute and chronic leukemias, and T-cell malignancies. Their uses are potentially unlimited in tumor imaging and in delivering cytotoxic agents to malignant cells. (For more details on monoclonal antibodies, see Chapter 7.)

Immune System

Antigens stimulate lymphokine release. In fact, excessive or scanty production of lymphokines may contribute to the development of disease, especially autoimmune or infectious diseases. Several types of lymphokines exist, including interleukins, interferons, and others.

Interleukins. Interleukins are divided into four groups: interleukin-1 (formerly called lymphocyte-activating factor), interleukin-2 (formerly called T-cell growth factor), interleukin-3, and interleukin-4 (also called B-cell stimulating factor 1).

Interleukin-1 (IL-1) exists in two structurally similar types: alpha and beta. Both types are produced by vascular tissues and almost all immune cells, including T cells, B cells, and NK cells. IL-1 production may be triggered by antigens, toxins, injury, or inflammation. This lymphokine acts as a cofactor during lymphocyte activation by promoting synthesis of other lymphokines and activating resting T cells. What's more, IL-1 combines with lymphokines that affect hematopoiesis (colony-stimulating factors), thus encouraging bone-marrow precursors to grow after their suppression by cytotoxic drugs.

IL-1 affects nonlymphoid tissues by:

- mediating the acute phase response, causing fever, hepatic protein synthesis, and release of neutrophils, adrenocorticotropic hormone, cortisol, and insulin
- promoting coagulation, leukocyte adherence, prostaglandin release, and hypotension through its effects on endothelial cells
- inducing formation of the enzyme protease and bone resorption, thereby possibly contributing to rheumatoid arthritis
- killing some tumor cells and insulin-producing beta cells.

IL-1 also possesses properties similar to those of tumor necrosis factor alpha.

Interleukin-2 (IL-2) initiates active T-cell proliferation, prompts synthesis of other lymphokines, and stimulates NK-cell growth. IL-2 also enhances the cytolytic activity of NK cells capable of killing tumor cells.

Produced by activated T cells, *interleukin-3 (IL-3)* is a colony-stimulating factor that affects hematopoiesis by encouraging growth of pluripotential stem cells. It's the growth factor for mast cells.

Interleukin-4 (IL-4) is the growth factor for activated B cells, resting T cells, and mast cells. It also enhances cytotoxic T-cell activity. After IL-4 prompts activated B cells to proliferate, another lymphokine—B-cell stimulating factor 2 or B-cell differentiating factor—prompts the proliferating B cells to become specialized immunoglobulin-secreting plasma cells.

Interferons. Produced in response to viral infection, these cells interfere with viral replication in infected cells. They have potent antiviral, antiproliferative, and immunologic properties. This group of lymphokines contains three main classes: alpha-interferon, beta-interferon, and gamma-interferon.

Alpha-interferon and *beta-interferon* both strengthen NK cell activity, increase Class I MHC molecules on lymphocytes, and regulate an-

Continued on page 14

Immune System

Antigen-presenting cells

Formed in the bone marrow, antigen-presenting cells (APCs) reside mainly in the skin, lymph nodes, spleen, and thymus. As their name suggests, they present antigens to antigen-sensitive lymphoid cells. The Langerhans' cell in the skin is the model APC.

APCs travel through the afferent lymphatics into the paracortex of draining lymph nodes. They interlock with many T cells, providing an efficient way to present antigens carried from the skin to T cells in the lymph nodes. APCs are rich in Class II MHC antigens (especially HLA-DR), which play a key role in presenting antigens to T cells. Other specialized APCs, called follicular dendritic cells, are located in the secondary follicles of the B-cell areas in the lymph nodes and spleen.

Lymphoid system cells—*continued*

tibody responses. However, their antiproliferative effects can make them immunosuppressive.

Gamma-interferon exerts many effects on the immune response and on nonlymphoid tissues. For instance, it induces Class I and Class II MHC molecules, activates macrophages, and interacts with other lymphokines. Gamma-interferon augments B cell–stimulating lymphokines and enhances antibody production, but it negates the effects of IL-1 on connective tissue by suppressing collagen synthesis.

Other lymphokines. Granulocyte-macrophage colony-stimulating factor influences the growth and differentiation of granulocyte and monocyte precursors. Two other lymphokines—tumor necrosis factor alpha (cachectin) and tumor necrosis factor beta (lymphotoxin)—are active in tumor necrosis, hypotension, inflammation, and several other biological responses.

Mononuclear phagocyte system

Formerly called the reticuloendothelial system, the mononuclear phagocyte system uses monocytes circulating in the bloodstream, which become macrophages in tissue. Mononuclear phagocytes play an important role in phagocytosis and in cell-mediated immunity because they're involved in initiating the immune response. (See *Antigen-presenting cells*.)

Polymorphonuclear granulocytes

Including neutrophils, eosinophils, basophils, and mast cells, polymorphonuclear granulocytes play a key role in phagocytosis. They also play a key role in acute inflammation and, teamed with antibodies and a series of sequentially reacting serum proteins (complement), help guard against foreign substances.

Platelets

Besides their coagulation function, platelets also take part in the immune response, especially in inflammation. They carry Class I MHC products and receptors for both IgG and IgE. After endothelial injury, platelets clump together at the endothelial surface and adhere there, releasing substances that increase permeability and activate complement components to attract leukocytes.

Immune response

When the immune system recognizes a foreign substance or antigen, it generally takes one of two courses of action. It may tolerate the antigen by *not* activating the immune response. Or it may respond to the antigen in an attempt to maintain homeostasis. (See *Encounter with an antigen*.) The immune system may respond either in a nonspecific or a specific way. (See *Understanding the immune response*, page 16.)

Immunologic tolerance

In immunologic tolerance, the immune system interprets a foreign antigen as a "self" antigen and may fail to direct a response against

Immune System

All about antigens

Usually a large protein or a form of protein, an antigen is any substance that elicits an immune response. Typically, it's not present in the body or exposed to the lymphoreticular system.

Recognizing an antigen and responding to it depends partly on the antigen's physical and chemical characteristics. However, the response also depends on the patient's genetic makeup and several other factors:
- *Age.* The immune system doesn't function as efficiently in infancy and in old age. In infancy, the specific immune system isn't completely developed; in the elderly, the immune state is hypofunctional, and specific immunologic functions decrease. Both age-groups may also have deficiencies in nonspecific immunity, such as thin skin and a poor inflammatory response.
- *Metabolism.* Some hormones affect the immune system. Adrenal and thyroid hormone deficiencies, for instance, increase susceptibility to infection. Steroid use inhibits phagocytosis and the inflammatory response, and also decreases humoral and cellular immunity.
- *Environment and lifestyle.* Poor living conditions and exposure to pathogens can increase susceptibility to infection. I.V. drug use and unsafe sexual practices can lead to such immune diseases as AIDS.
- *Nutrition.* Poor nutrition in infancy can thwart development of the immune response, especially cell-mediated immunity, leading to recurrent infections of the GI and respiratory tracts, for example.
- *Skin and mucous membrane condition.* These are the body's first line of defense against invasion by foreign substances. These tissues act in nonspecific immunity by providing a physical barrier to invasion. Damage increases their susceptibility to infection.
- *Microbial flora.* The body's normal microbial flora helps in developing natural antibodies to certain organisms. It also suppresses overgrowth of pathogenic and possibly virulent organisms.
- *Physiologic activity.* Cilia action in the respiratory tract, normal urine flow, skin secretions, and enzyme activity aid in normal immune function.

Encounter with an antigen

This diagram shows the possible outcomes of a host's encounter with an antigen.

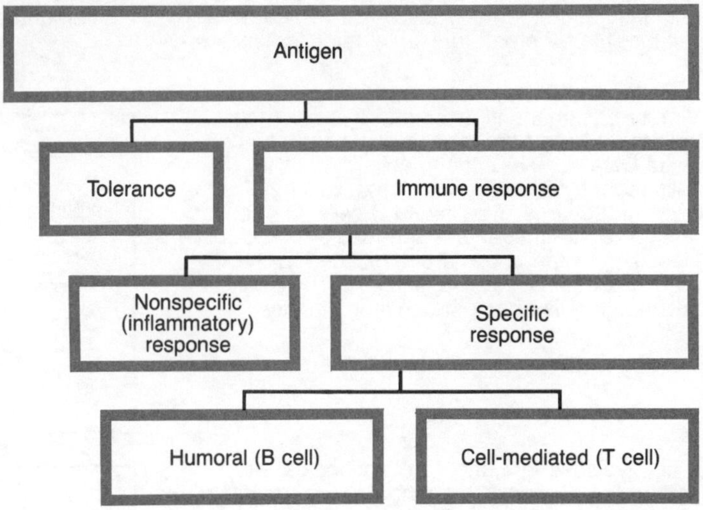

that specific antigen. Because tolerance is antigen-specific, tolerance to one antigen doesn't suggest tolerance to any others.

Why would the immune system tolerate a foreign substance? Immunologic immaturity may be one reason. Others include the host's genetic makeup and the complexity, persistence, distribution, dose, and administration route of the particular antigen.

Nonspecific immune responses

A nonspecific response occurs when the host encounters a foreign substance and then reacts in the same way at each subsequent encounter. (See *Comparing encounters with an antigen*, page 17.) Two nonspecific responses, inflammation and phagocytosis, eliminate most foreign substances.

Inflammation. The body's response to tissue injury, inflammation involves movement of phagocytes into the affected area to restore homeostasis. (See *Signs and symptoms of inflammation*, page 17.) Three main events occur during inflammation:
- Blood supply increases to the affected area.
- Capillary permeability increases because of endothelial cell retraction. This permits large molecules to pass across the endothelium, allowing the soluble mediators of immunity to reach the site.
- Phagocytes move from the capillaries to the surrounding tissues and finally to the site.

Phagocytes localize and remove foreign substances from the body by a carefully orchestrated process. First, the cells must travel to the inflammation site in a process called chemotaxis. Once there, chemotactic peptides (complement components, especially C5a) are released. These peptides enter the capillaries bordering the inflammation site, causing phagocytic cells (especially neutrophils) to adhere to the capillary endothelium. Then the phagocytes leave the vessel, traveling up the concentration gradient of the chemotactic peptides toward the inflammation site.

Continued on page 16

Immune System

Understanding the immune response

The immune response represents the body's way of recognizing and destroying antigens. Its primary weapons are T cells and B cells. T cells interact directly with an antigen to provide cellular immunity and stop neoplastic growth. They're also responsible for organ transplant rejection and certain autoimmune disorders. B cells incite production of immunoglobulins, which attack antigens. These immunoglobulins include IgM, IgG, IgA, IgD, and IgE. The following diagrams show how the immune system works.

Viral or bacterial antigens adhere to cell membranes, escape from their protein coats, and release DNA or RNA into the cell's cytoplasm. The cells react by releasing interferon, which helps inactivate the virus. T cells and B cells interact and recognize the antigen through markers on its surface. The lymph nodes are stimulated by the thymus to release T cells sensitized to the particular antigen. T cells attack the antigen directly.

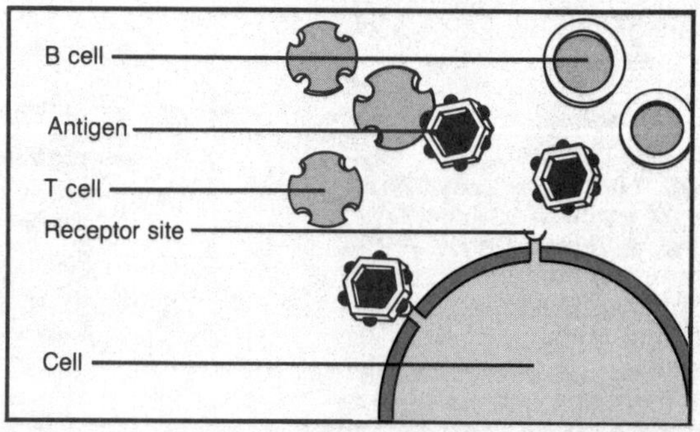

B cells release IgM, then IgG antibodies, which adhere to specific sites on the antigen's surface. This attachment causes antibody shape to change and activates circulating proteins in a process called the complement cascade. Complement stimulates histamine, prostaglandin, and bradykinin release, increasing capillary permeability, vasodilation, and macrophage release.

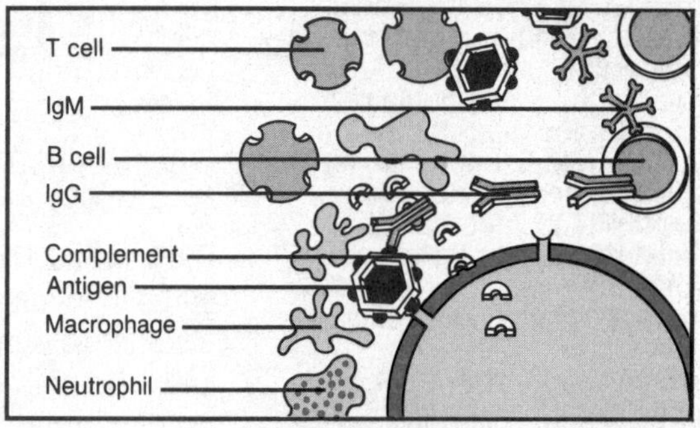

Complement roughens the antigen's surface, giving it a positive charge. This attracts macrophages and neutrophils, which engulf and attack the cell. Lysosomes adhere to the cell and release hydrolase, an enzyme that breaks down the cells' protein and lipids. Some IgGs return to lymphoid tissue and remain dormant until the antigen reappears. These antibodies remember the antigen, resulting in a rapid, intensified second immune response and long-term immunity.

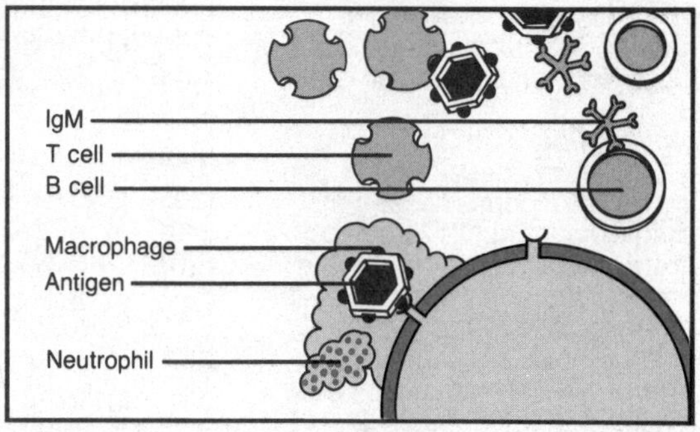

Immune response—*continued*

Phagocytosis. This process takes place when the phagocytes reach the inflammation site. After recognizing the foreign substance, they attach to and engulf it. (See *A look at phagocytes,* page 18.)

During the attachment phase, phagocytes adhere to the foreign substance using one of two methods. The first employs nonspecific cell-surface receptors. The second method, called opsonization, employs antibody coating of the foreign substance, enhancing the phagocyte's ability to bind to it.

Ingestion occurs next. First, the phagocyte surrounds the foreign substance by wrapping it in pseudopods. Then the phagocyte takes the foreign substance into the cytoplasm and closes it inside a

Immune System

phagosome (vacuole.) Next, lysosomes fuse with the phagosome, destroying the foreign substance. If the substance is a microorganism, undigested microbial products may be released outside the cell.

Many unencapsulated bacteria are quickly taken up by phagocytes and destroyed. However, encapsulated strains such as *Pneumococcus* may resist phagocytosis and avoid destruction.

Specific immune responses

A specific response occurs when the host encounters a foreign substance and reacts to it, creating antibodies or a cell-mediated response designed to dispose of the invader.

Specific immune responses differ from nonspecific ones not only in their specificity but also in their heterogeneity and memory. *Specificity* describes the way in which components of the immune response react only with antigens that are identical or similar to those that started the response. *Heterogeneity* indicates that various cell types and products interact in different ways. *Memory* means that each subsequent exposure to a specific antigen triggers a magnified and accelerated immune response.

Two effector mechanisms control specific immune responses: humoral immunity (mediated by antibodies) and cell-mediated immunity (mediated by specifically sensitized lymphocytes).

Humoral immunity. Also called antibody-mediated immunity, humoral immunity is controlled by B cells. Extracellular or cell-bound antibodies produced by B cells and plasma react with the antigen that spurred their production. B cells activate production of antibodies that then attack the antigen, causing the antigen to bind with an antibody.

How, though, do B cells produce antibodies? To begin, IgM or IgD immunoglobulins on the B-cell surface recognize the antigen. Once this occurs, resting B cells increase their cytoplasmic volume, entering the early phase of cell cycling, and become more receptive to other cell-activation cues. These cues include the B-cell growth and differentiation factors created by T cells. T-helper cells signal B cells to activate, usually promoted by contact between B cells and T-helper cells. What's more, T-helper cells become active when they encounter antigens on antigen-presenting cells.

Other humoral factors can also intensify the immune response without cell participation. The *complement system* is the best example of this. The main humoral mediator in antigen-antibody reactions, the complement system has three main functions:

- It covers pathogenic organisms or immune complexes with opsonins, promoting ingestion of the particle by phagocytes (opsonic function).
- It stimulates inflammatory cells, such as granulocytes and lymphocytes, binding them to specific receptors and causing responses such as chemotaxis (inflammatory function).
- It destroys target cells—viruses, bacteria, fungi, parasites, virus-infected cells, and tumor cells—through the macromolecular membrane attack complex formed by complement proteins (cytotoxic function).

Continued on page 18

Comparing encounters with an antigen

When an antigen invades the body for the first time, the body usually attempts to eliminate it by phagocytosis. Many factors influence the effectiveness of phagocytosis, including the host's general health and the amount and type of antigen.

If phagocytosis succeeds, the antigen is eliminated and disease symptoms, if seen, will be minimal at most. However, if it fails, the disease may occur or progress. At this point, antibodies step in. Now the disease's course depends on the efficiency of antibody production and cell-mediated immunity. Once antibody appears and complement promotes uptake of an encapsulated antigen, phagocytes can kill the invader. What's more, phagocytosis intensifies and the antigen can be eliminated when cell-mediated immunity starts and effector molecules are produced.

This process intensifies during all subsequent encounters with the antigen. Each time the body recognizes the antigen, it produces more cells involved in humoral or cell-mediated immunity.

However, underlying disease, immunosuppressants, or a massive dose of challenge inoculum can inhibit the immune response even on subsequent encounters. In such cases, the outcome depends on whether phagocytosis and the inflammatory response can remove the antigen with little or no help from humoral or cell-mediated immunity.

Signs and symptoms of inflammation

Inflammation's classic signs include redness, warmth, swelling, pain, and loss of function. Redness and warmth result from increased perfusion caused by the vasodilative effects of histamine or kinins released at the injury site. Swelling occurs when serum leaks from the capillaries into the tissues, whereas pain arises when nerve endings are irritated by bradykinin, a chemical mediator, or are subject to increased pressure from swelling. Loss of function results from swelling and pain.

Immune System

A look at phagocytes

Phagocytes engulf other cells and foreign particles—a process known as phagocytosis. Phagocytes include mononuclear phagocytes, neutrophils, eosinophils, and mediator cells.

Mononuclear phagocytes
The mononuclear phagocyte system (MPS), formerly called the reticuloendothelial system, includes circulating monocytes, which become the macrophages found in tissues. These cells disseminate throughout the body, eliminating foreign substances from the blood, lymph, and tissue. Through a process called endocytosis, they remove and destroy some types of bacteria; damaged, worn-out, or neoplastic cells; colloidal materials; and macromolecules. The MPS probably plays a crucial role in first recognizing an antigen.

Neutrophils
Also called polymorphonuclear leukocytes, neutrophils break down ingested material and kill foreign substances, such as microorganisms.

Eosinophils
Although no one knows the eosinophils' precise role in phagocytosis, we do know that they can envelop and destroy microorganisms, soluble antigen-antibody complexes, and many other kinds of particles. What's more, they probably ingest immune complexes and limit inflammatory reactions by antagonizing the effects of certain mediators. They may also participate in tissue injury (possibly by releasing toxic components) and may take part in antibody-mediated cytotoxic reactions that are important in clearing some parasites.

Mediator cells
These cells engage in various immunologic activities, such as releasing chemical substances that increase vascular permeability, cause smooth muscle contraction, and enhance the inflammatory response. Mediator cells include mast cells, basophils, platelets, and enterochromaffin cells. Basophils and platelets, the major mediator cells in the circulatory system, contain several vasoactive amines, including histamine and serotonin.

Immune response—*continued*

The complement system contains at least 20 separate plasma proteins. Appearing in the bloodstream as inactive molecules, these proteins must undergo sequential activation before a complement reaction can progress.

Complement activation can take place through classic or alternative pathways. (See *Complement pathways*.) The *classic pathway* may be immunologically triggered by antigen-antibody (immune) complexes or by IgG, IgG_2, IgG_3, or IgM. It can also be nonimmunologically triggered by C-reactive protein, DNA, trypsin-like enzymes, staphylococcal protein A, retrovirus, cardiac mitochondrial membranes, polynucleotides, or urate crystals. Usually, activation takes place when any of these substances bind directly with the C1 component.

The *alternative pathway* can be stimulated by C3b or by substances that prevent inactivation of the enzyme C3bBb. Other trigger substances include polysaccharides, yeast cell walls, bacterial cell-wall components, viruses, parasites, fungi, certain tumor cells, cobra venom factor, nephritic factor, radiographic contrast media, and dialysis membranes.

Both the classic and alternative pathways proceed sequentially through three phases: initiation, amplification, and membrane attack. Recognition of a foreign substance initiates the pathway. Amplification involves the action of proteases and additional molecules. Finally, membrane attack occurs and the cell dies.

If uncontrolled, the effects of the complement system could be dangerous even to host cells. So the immune system attempts to limit complement's effects to the local site. If it fails to do so, complement may contribute to disease or to immune complex formation.

In some cases, autoantibodies are involved in abnormal complement effects and arise with tissue damage or infection. When an autoantibody binds with a complement element, it may turn the complement system against the host's own tissue. This occurs in such disorders as Goodpasture's syndrome, myasthenia gravis, and rheumatic myocarditis.

Tissue injury, inflammation, and vasculitis can occur when immune complexes activate complement in the walls of small vessels and capillaries. Called the Arthus reaction, this process causes serum sickness and hypersensitivity pneumonitis. Circulating immune complexes are found in a variety of diseases, including infections, neoplasms, and autoimmune disorders.

A lack of complement components—either congenital or acquired—can also cause disease. Genetic deficiencies usually occur in the C2 component, but deficiencies in C8 (causing increased susceptibility to *Neisseria* infections) and C3 and C5 (causing pyrogenic infections) also occur. Acquired deficiencies involve circulating immune complexes, giving rise to connective tissue disorders, such as systemic lupus erythematosus.

Other humoral factors associated with the immune response include the kallikrein system and slow-reacting substance of anaphylaxis. The kallikrein system consists of plasma proteins activated by an

Continued on page 20

Immune System

Complement pathways

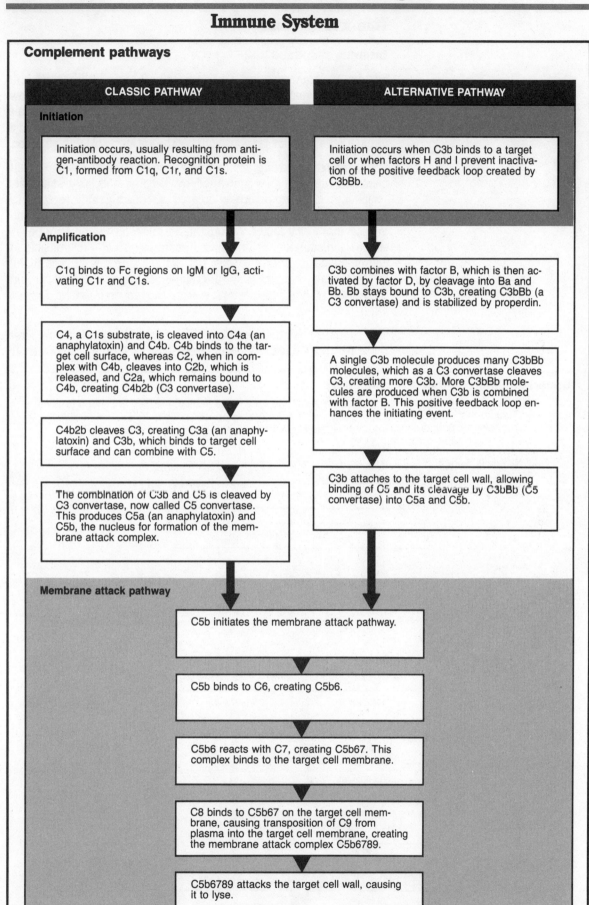

CLASSIC PATHWAY	ALTERNATIVE PATHWAY

Initiation

Classic pathway: Initiation occurs, usually resulting from antigen-antibody reaction. Recognition protein is C1, formed from C1q, C1r, and C1s.

Alternative pathway: Initiation occurs when C3b binds to a target cell or when factors H and I prevent inactivation of the positive feedback loop created by C3bBb.

Amplification

Classic pathway:

C1q binds to Fc regions on IgM or IgG, activating C1r and C1s.

C4, a C1s substrate, is cleaved into C4a (an anaphylatoxin) and C4b. C4b binds to the target cell surface, whereas C2, when in complex with C4b, cleaves into C2b, which is released, and C2a, which remains bound to C4b, creating C4b2b (C3 convertase).

C4b2b cleaves C3, creating C3a (an anaphylatoxin) and C3b, which binds to target cell surface and can combine with C5.

The combination of C3b and C5 is cleaved by C3 convertase, now called C5 convertase. This produces C5a (an anaphylatoxin) and C5b, the nucleus for formation of the membrane attack complex.

Alternative pathway:

C3b combines with factor B, which is then activated by factor D, by cleavage into Ba and Bb. Bb stays bound to C3b, creating C3bBb (a C3 convertase) and is stabilized by properdin.

A single C3b molecule produces many C3bBb molecules, which as a C3 convertase cleaves C3, creating more C3b. More C3bBb molecules are produced when C3b is combined with factor B. This positive feedback loop enhances the initiating event.

C3b attaches to the target cell wall, allowing binding of C5 and its cleavage by C3bBb (C5 convertase) into C5a and C5b.

Membrane attack pathway

C5b initiates the membrane attack pathway.

C5b binds to C6, creating C5b6.

C5b6 reacts with C7, creating C5b67. This complex binds to the target cell membrane.

C8 binds to C5b67 on the target cell membrane, causing transposition of C9 from plasma into the target cell membrane, creating the membrane attack complex C5b6789.

C5b6789 attacks the target cell wall, causing it to lyse.

Immune System

Immune response—*continued*

antigen-antibody reaction. The enzyme kallikrein interacts with its substrate to create vasoactive peptides, such as bradykinins. Slow-reacting substance of anaphylaxis is released when antigen interacts with sensitized cells. Certain coagulation proteins may also intensify the immune response during the antigen-antibody reaction.

Cell-mediated immunity. Reflecting a specific immune response, cell-mediated immunity is controlled by T cells, specially sensitized lymphocytes, or lymphokines created when antigens interact with specially sensitized lymphocytes. These lymphokines include migration inhibitory factor, cytotoxin, and interferon and may be the effector molecules of cell-mediated immunity. T cells responsible for cell-mediated immunity attack the antigen directly by functioning as killer cells, indirectly by functioning as helper cells, or through the action of lymphokines. (See *Understanding cell-mediated immunity*.)

How do cell-mediated reactions differ from humoral ones? First, these reactions have a delayed onset; that's why they're sometimes

Understanding cell-mediated immunity

Cell-mediated responses occur after antigen presentation and T-cell activation. This activation is controlled by T-suppressor and T-helper cells. T cells called macrophage-activating cells, through their effects on lymphokines, activate macrophages to intensify their phagocytic and bactericidal roles. T-cytotoxic cells, activated by antigen, receive support from T-helper cells. These helper cells also work with B cells to produce antibody that activates cells, such as killer (K) cells, carrying Fc receptors. Natural killer (NK) cells work nonspecifically, especially against cellular targets.

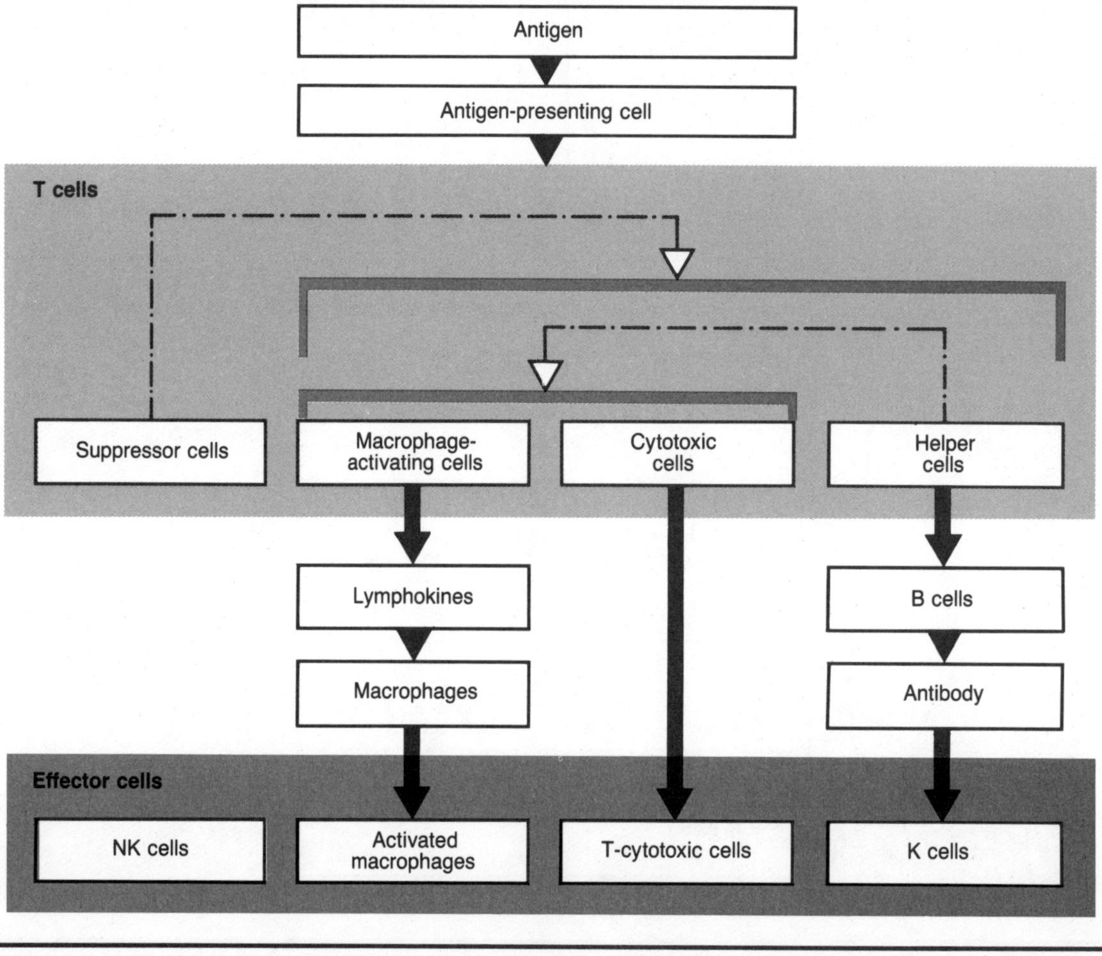

Immune System

Immunopotentiation and immunosuppression

In immunopotentiation, an intrinsic or extrinsic factor magnifies the immune response. Changing just one step in the chain of immunologic reactions can enhance this response by:

- reducing the response's "latent" period
- intensifying the response
- lengthening its duration
- causing a response to an antigen that previously didn't elicit one.

Immunopotentiation occurs in both humoral and cell-mediated immunity. However, a substance that enhances a response in one system might suppress it in another. Two types of immunopotentiators enhance the immune response: *nonspecific immunopotentiators* (also called adjuvants), which increase humoral and cell-mediated responses to many different antigens, and *specific immunopotentiators*, which enhance the response to a small group of antigens. Vaccines are a common type of immunopotentiator.

Immunosuppression can have positive or negative effects on the host. It can result from normal immunoregulatory mechanisms, underlying disease, disordered immunoregulation, or exogenous factors, such as drugs. (See Chapter 7 for more details).

called delayed hypersensitivity reactions. Second, these reactions need living lymphocytes or their products to evoke the immune response. And third, these reactions involve low-weight sensitized lymphocytes (effector cells.) Cell-mediated reactions seem to be particularly effective against cell-bound antigens or those otherwise inaccessible to antibodies.

A cell-mediated reaction is initiated when an antigen binds with an antigen receptor on the surface of a sensitized T cell. Although this can occur directly, it's usually mediated by macrophage-bound antigen in association with "self" determinants or other substances. Once this takes place, T-helper or T-suppressor cells are generated for T-T and T-B interactions. T-cytotoxic cells, T cells that enhance effector cells controlling cell-mediated immunity, and memory cells are also generated.

T-helper cells and macrophages are instrumental in triggering a cell-mediated immune response. To initiate the response, an antigen-presenting cell such as a macrophage activates the small number of T-helper cells that have antigen-specific receptors by presenting the antigen to the T cells along with "self" MHC molecules. Activated T-helper cells produce lymphokines, such as IL-1 and IL-2, that activate macrophages and attract other lymphocytes and macrophages to take part in the response. Macrophage activation factor is released to enhance macrophage function. Activated macrophages secrete IL-1 along with several enzymes that can digest connective tissue, procoagulant molecules that prompt local coagulation through the extrinsic coagulation pathway, and a plasminogen activator that changes plasminogen to plasmin. Plasmin digests fibrin and slowly reverses clot formation.

Other lymphokines are also released. Macrophage chemotactic factor mobilizes cells to the reaction site and migration inhibition factor immobilizes macrophages and localizes them near the site. Release of macrophage aggregation factor helps the cells adhere to each other.

T-helper cells release IL-2 to activate T-suppressor cells, which control the functions of both T cells and B cells, usually by suppressor factors that block T-helper cell activity and B-cell differentiation into plasma cells. T-cytotoxic cells function in transplant rejections and tumor cell destruction.

Helper and suppressor T-cell functions must be balanced to regulate all the immunoglobulin isotypes. Sometimes, IL-1 is also necessary for B-cell activation. Immunoglobulin synthesis progresses once B cells differentiate into plasma cells. After a sensitized lymphocyte interacts with an immunoglobulin, the lymphocyte can act.

Development of immune-mediated disease

After encountering a foreign substance, the body undergoes a period of disequilibrium. Usually, the immune system responds appropriately, restoring immunologic balance. But suppose the immune response is inappropriate or its components function incorrectly. Then immunologic imbalance—and immune-mediated disease—will result. (See *Immunopotentiation and immunosuppression*.)

The following four chapters discuss diseases caused by immunologic dysfunction.

Immune System

Self-Test

1. B cells are the primary mediators of:
a. inflammation **b.** phagocytosis **c.** humoral immunity **d.** cell-mediated immunity

2. T-helper (T-inducer) cells may also be referred to as:
a. CD4 cells **b.** CD8 cells **c.** TH_1 cells **d.** TI_1 cells

3. All of the following occur during inflammation except:
a. capillary permeability increases **b.** blood supply increases to the affected area **c.** phagocytes move from the capillaries into the surrounding tissue **d.** phagocytes attach to and engulf the foreign substance

4. Complement is associated with:
a. inflammation **b.** phagocytosis **c.** humoral immunity **d.** cell-mediated immunity

5. T cells responsible for cell-mediated immunity attack the antigen by all of the following except:
a. directly, by functioning as immunoglobulins **b.** through the action of lymphokines **c.** directly, by functioning as killer cells **d.** indirectly, by functioning as helper cells

6. The main serum immunoglobulin is:
a. IgG **b.** IgA **c.** IgM **d.** IgE

7. The immunoglobulin associated with immediate hypersensitivity reactions is:
a. IgG **b.** IgA **c.** IgM **d.** IgE

8. Secondary lymphoid structures include all of the following except:
a. spleen **b.** lymph nodes **c.** bone marrow **d.** mucosal-associated lymphoid tissue

9. The α/β heterodimer of the T cell's CD molecule recognizes viral antigens along with:
a. Class I MHC molecules **b.** Class II MHC molecules **c.** Class III MHC molecules **d.** Class IV MHC molecules

10. Immunoglobulin is produced by:
a. T-helper cells **b.** T-suppressor cells **c.** plasma cells **d.** memory B cells

Answers (page number shows where answer appears in text)
1. **c** (page 17) 2. **a** (page 7) 3. **d** (page 15) 4. **c** (page 17) 5. **a** (page 20) 6. **a** (page 11) 7. **d** (page 12) 8. **c** (page 5) 9. **a** (page 9) 10. **c** (page 9)

Autoimmune Disorders: When Immunity Goes Awry

JoAnn B. Reckling and **Geri Budesheim Neuberger** wrote this chapter. Both women work at the University of Kansas in Kansas City. Ms. Reckling is a research assistant and Dr. Neuberger is an associate professor of medical-surgical nursing.

Autoimmune disorders occur when the body's immune system produces antibodies that act on normal endogenous antigens. Called autoantibodies, these antibodies carry out the immune response on normal body cells and, consequently, cause varying degrees of tissue damage. Depending on the severity of the autoimmune response, tissue damage ranges from minor local effects to potentially life-threatening systemic ones.

Autoimmune disorders may be classified as organ-specific or organ-nonspecific (systemic). Organ-specific disorders involve autoimmune responses to antigens in a specific organ. Examples include type I diabetes mellitus, Hashimoto's thyroiditis, and myasthenia gravis. Organ-nonspecific autoimmune disorders involve autoimmune responses to widespread self-antigenic cells, tissues, or both. In these disorders, immune complex deposition occurs throughout the body, especially in the kidneys, joints, and skin. Examples include systemic lupus erythematosus, rheumatoid arthritis, progressive systemic sclerosis (or scleroderma), Goodpasture's syndrome, polymyositis, and dermatomyositis. More than one autoimmune disorder may occur simultaneously.

In this chapter, we'll start with a general review of autoimmune disorders. Later, we'll detail some of the specific disorders you're most likely to encounter.

Understanding autoimmune dysfunction

Although not entirely understood, autoantibody production apparently results from the immune system's inability to distinguish between self and nonself, thereby disrupting tolerance to self. (See *Recognition of self,* and *Tolerance: Forgiving immunity,* page 24.) At their root, autoimmune disorders may result from a complex interplay of immunologic, genetic, hormonal, virologic, and other factors.

Immunologic factors may include:
- release of sequestered antigens
- diminished T-suppressor cell function
- lack of tolerance at the T-cell level and antigenic mimicry
- thymic defects
- exogenous polyclonal B-cell activators
- macrophage defects
- aberrant expression of class II major histocompatibility complex (MHC) antigens
- defective tolerance induction
- pluripotential stem cell defects
- defects in production of and response to accessory signals for B-cell proliferation and differentiation
- lymphokine defects, especially involving interleukins
- defects in the idiotype–anti-idiotype network and idiotype mimicry of autoantigen.

Genetic factors play a role in determining the incidence, onset, and nature of the autoimmune response. The MHC genes—especially the DR2, DR3, DR4, and DR5 alleles—and genes that code for antigen receptors on B cells and T cells apparently participate.

Continued on page 24

Recognition of self

A central mechanism of immunity, recognition of self primarily involves the responses of T and B cells to the body's own major histocompatibility complex antigens. These responses initiate and regulate both humoral and cellular immunity through complex, highly organized interactions of complementary T-cell and B-cell surface-bound and soluble idiotypes (single antigens or groups of antigens that distinguish among different immunoglobulin molecules) and anti-idiotypes (antibodies that act against these idiotypes).

The body's immune system reacts to antigenic determinants, or epitopes, through antigen-combining sites in the V (variable) regions of immunoglobulins that are either secreted by or located on the surfaces of lymphocytes. In a given immunoglobulin, the V region itself can act as an epitope, generating a new set of antibodies that recognize a particular immunoglobulin as distinct from others. Each antibody molecule acts to recognize a given antigen, then in turn becomes antigenic itself.

Both T cells and B cells, along with their soluble products (such as antibodies and antigen-specific T-helper and T-suppressor cells), express idiotypic determinants. In addition, the idiotype of immunoglobulin secreted by an antibody-forming B cell is similar to that of the cell surface immunoglobulin receptors for antigen.

Autoimmune Disorders

Tolerance: Forgiving immunity

Tolerance refers to the immune system's ability to recognize and not react to self antigens. This ability is apparently acquired during fetal development from direct contact between self components and specific antigen-reactive cells.

Tolerance is classified as central or peripheral. In central tolerance, several mechanisms may contribute to the lack of immune response. In the first, called *clonal deletion*, fetal T-cell and B-cell clones are eliminated by direct contact with their specific autoantigens. In *clonal anergy* or abortion, antigen-binding B cells are unable to react to antigen. Finally, in *antigen-induced inactivation*, lymphocytes lose their reactivity through an interaction between antigenic determinants and cell surface receptors that bind such determinants.

In peripheral tolerance, some antibody is produced initially. However, T-suppressor cells, antibodies, anti-idiotypes, and immune complexes rapidly reduce or halt antibody production.

These mechanisms aren't necessarily mutually exclusive. Several may occur simultaneously, producing different degrees or types of tolerance.

Continued

Autoimmune disorders frequently accompany deficiencies in certain complement components. The X chromosome has been implicated because many of these disorders affect more women than men. However, this association may be hormonally related.

Hormonal factors are suspected because some autoimmune disorders affect one sex more than the other. Connective tissue disease, for instance, strikes more women than men, whereas ankylosing spondylitis affects more men than women. Evidence of hormonal involvement comes from the known action of pituitary, thyroid, parathyroid, adrenal, and gonadal hormones in the immune response. Researchers are now investigating the immunosuppressive effects of testosterone and the immunoenhancing effects of estrogen.

Viruses are often implicated as the cause of autoimmune disorders or a contributing factor to them. These include the Epstein-Barr virus, myxoviruses, hepatitis viruses, cytomegaloviruses, coxsackieviruses, and retroviruses. Most of these viruses can induce both autoantibody production during active infection and autoimmune-like characteristics, such as vasculitis and glomerulonephritis. However, these disease characteristics may result from virus–viral antibody complexes rather than from autoantibody-antigen complexes.

Autoimmune disorders may also be related to lymph tissue hyperplasia, malignant proliferation of lymphocytes or plasma cells, and such immunodeficiencies as hypogammaglobulinemia, selective IgA deficiency, and complement deficiencies. Autoantibodies also sometimes develop as part of aging.

Pathophysiology. In autoimmune dysfunction, the pathophysiology of tissue damage is understood somewhat better than the cause. Three primary mechanisms seem to mediate the abnormal autoimmune response. (See *Immunopathologic mechanisms in autoimmune disease*.)

Assessment

The insidious and unpredictable nature of autoimmune disorders will challenge your assessment skills. Detection of these disorders requires careful evaluation of signs and symptoms and diagnostic test results.

Assessment of patients with possible autoimmune disorders requires a complete history and physical examination. Focus the health history on areas related to autoimmune disorders. For instance, because genetic factors seem to play an important role in autoimmune dysfunction, be sure to explore family health history. And because certain drugs can stimulate an autoimmune response, ask about the patient's current drug use.

During the physical examination, keep in mind that some autoimmune disorders, such as Hashimoto's thyroiditis, typically affect particular target organs. Conversely, other autoimmune disorders tend to cause systemic signs, such as fever, fatigue, weakness, joint pain and stiffness, and rashes. Be alert for signs and symptoms of inflammation—redness, heat, swelling, pain, and loss of function in the joints, skin, or other areas of the body.

Autoimmune Disorders

Immunopathologic mechanisms in autoimmune disease

Three basic mechanisms mediate the immune response to autoantibodies, as shown in the chart below.

Mechanism	Features	Associated autoimmune disorders
Antibody action on cell surface structures	• Usually destroys cells or tissues. • May stimulate or inhibit certain cell functions without causing cell destruction. • Complement or antibody (or both) contributes to cytotoxicity.	• Autoimmune hemolytic anemias, neutropenias, lymphopenias, and thrombocytopenias (occurring either independently or in such disorders as systemic lupus erythematosus and rheumatoid arthritis) • Anti-glomerular basement membrane antibody-induced conditions, such as Goodpasture's syndrome • Autoimmune endocrinopathies, such as Hashimoto's thyroiditis, type I diabetes mellitus, and Addison's disease • Antireceptor-mediated diseases, such as Graves' disease and myasthenia gravis
Antigen-antibody (immune) complexes in intercellular fluid or in circulation	• Immune complexes are deposited in tissues with large filtering membranes, such as the kidneys, joints, and the choroid plexus. • Complement factors and granulocytic and monocytic cells are attracted to sites of complex deposition. • Cell death follows.	• Glomerulonephritis • Systemic lupus erythematosus • Rheumatoid arthritis
Sensitized T cells	• Tissue lesions, probably produced by release of lymphokines.	• Several disorders in association with the two mechanisms listed above, such as sarcoidosis

Diagnostic tests. Key tests used to detect autoimmune disorders include blood studies, urinalysis, and tests for autoantibodies and autoimmune reaction products.

The complete blood count (CBC) and routine urinalysis help screen for an autoimmune disorder. Reduced levels of CBC components may result if antibodies (such as antiplatelet antibodies) exist to destroy them or if an immune problem prevents their adequate production. Hematuria or proteinuria can result from glomerular damage such as that caused by immune complex deposition. Although such findings by themselves will not confirm an autoimmune disorder, they do indicate the need for further testing.

After initial screening, immunologic tests may be performed to detect autoantibodies or other abnormal autoimmune cellular functions. Assays for T cells and B cells may be performed on tissue sections or on fresh suspensions of cells from blood, bone marrow, or other organs. However, these assays can only classify immunocompetent cells; lymphocyte function must be evaluated to reveal autoimmune dysfunction.

Other diagnostic studies aim to detect an abnormal antibody level or type or an abnormal amount of an immune function product, such as complement.

- *Immunoprecipitation (immunoelectrophoresis)* uses standard amounts of antigen and antibody to measure the serum level of an unknown antigen. The test can measure complement components, serum immunoglobulins, and some other serum proteins.
- *Agglutination tests* measure concentrations or titers of antigen rather than actual amounts of antigen. In these tests, mixing a particulate antigen with its antibody causes cells to clump together

Continued on page 26

Autoimmune Disorders

Continued

and sink to the bottom of the test tube, an observable finding that verifies a reaction (or absence of a reaction) to a specific antibody.

- In *immunofluorescence tests*, antibody molecules are treated with fluorescent dyes that do not interfere with molecular function. The reaction of these treated antibody molecules to antigen-containing cells or tissues produces a visible fluorescent-stained immune complex.
- *Radioimmunoassay* can determine the level of any small molecule that stimulates antibody production. The test involves mixing a known quantity of radioisotope-tagged antigen and its specific antibody with a serum sample. If the sample also contains the antigen, some of that antigen will bind with the antibody in the solution, displacing some of the radioisotope-tagged antigen. Measuring the radioactivity of the antigen-antibody complexes formed and comparing the results with known standards indicate the amount of complexes formed from antigen in the sample and the amount formed from radioisotope-tagged antigen complexing with the antibody.
- *Complement assays* measure levels of complement and its components. These tests are based on complement's ability to destroy sensitized red blood cells. Reduced levels may indicate that an autoimmune disorder is consuming available complement and using it to form antibody-antigen complexes. Elevated levels may indicate increased complement production.
- *Organ or tissue biopsies* are often required to confirm diagnosis. Skin lesion biopsy may reveal vasculitis or immune complex deposition. Renal biopsy may enable identification of an autoimmune process affecting the glomeruli. Liver biopsy provides definitive diagnosis of autoimmune liver disease.

The following pages review selected organ-specific and organ-nonspecific disorders, including systemic lupus erythematosus, rheumatoid arthritis, and others.

Systemic lupus erythematosus

Systemic lupus erythematosus (SLE) is a multisystem disorder characterized by the presence of various autoantibodies. SLE occurs most frequently in women during the second to fifth decades of life, but also occurs in children and the elderly. It has a higher incidence among nonwhites—especially among blacks. Its course varies widely; some patients have little involvement, whereas others have life-threatening problems. Also, the disease may follow an erratic course that includes spontaneous remissions and exacerbations.

The exact cause of SLE remains unclear, but altered immune responsiveness seems to play an important role, as evidenced by increased B-cell and decreased T-suppressor cell activity. Many factors influence development of SLE. The most striking is diffuse production of autoantibodies. In fact, the patient may have autoantibodies to red blood cells, neutrophils, platelets, lymphocytes, or almost any organ or tissue in the body.

Genetic factors probably participate as well; SLE patients have an increased frequency of HLA-DR2 and HLA-DR3 antigens. These patients also seem to have an inherited deficiency in cell surface

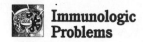

Autoimmune Disorders

Drug-induced lupus syndrome

In susceptible patients, certain drugs can produce a lupus-like syndrome, including arthralgias, arthritis, rash, and possibly fever and pleurisy. Discontinuing drug therapy usually causes disease remission.

Many drugs have been implicated in this syndrome, including:
- acebutolol
- aminoglutethimide
- aminosalicylic acid
- chlorpromazine
- griseofulvin
- hydralazine
- isoniazid
- levodopa
- mephenytoin
- methyldopa
- methylthiouracil
- oral contraceptives
- penicillamine
- penicillin
- phenylbutazone
- phenytoin
- pindolol
- procainamide
- propylthiouracil
- streptomycin
- sulfonamides
- tetracyclines
- trimethadione

C3b receptors. Hormonal factors also contribute; women are far more susceptible to the disease than men, and many suffer exacerbation during pregnancy or the postpartum period. Environmental factors are also important; SLE may flare after viral infection, exposure to ultraviolet light, surgery, or stress. (See *Drug-induced lupus syndrome*.)

Tissue injury in SLE results from autoantibody activity and immune complex deposition at various sites. The disease has no characteristic clinical pattern, and all organ systems may be involved. Inflammatory tissue changes may include edema, extravasation of red blood cells, cell destruction, fibrin deposition, and cell membrane thickening. Immunoglobulin and complement deposition may occur at such points as the epidermal-dermal junction in the skin and along the kidney's basement membrane.

Specific immunologic features of SLE include:
- lupus erythematosus (LE) cell. This is formed when nuclei sensitized to nucleoprotein are phagocytized by polymorphonuclear leukocytes.
- antinuclear antibodies (ANA). High ANA titers are most often associated with SLE. Antibodies to single- and double-stranded DNA and to the Smith (Sm) antigen are also characteristic.
- immune complexes (antigen-antibody formation). Immune complex deposition initiates complement-mediated tissue injury in SLE. Although immune complexes can be detected in SLE patients, they're not specific for the disease. In fact, immune complexes appear in most rheumatic and many nonrheumatic diseases.
- reduced complement levels. These may stem from decreased complement component production, increased complement use by immune complexes, or a combination of both.
- tissue deposition of immunoglobulins and complement. This takes place along the glomerular basement membrane and at the epidermal-dermal junction.
- circulating anticoagulants. Prolonged thromboplastin and partial thromboplastin times may indicate the presence of antibodies to circulating anticoagulants. Patients with these antibodies are at an increased risk for venous thrombi and, if pregnant, for miscarriages.

SLE's course and prognosis vary greatly. The disease may run a mild course or may become severe and fatal. Complications of therapy—including atherosclerosis, infection, and cancer—are common causes of death.

Assessment

Because SLE can produce diverse, widely varying features, you'll need to take a complete health history and perform a physical examination. During the history, be alert for complaints of fatigue, malaise, fever, rash, and weight loss. Because the disease shows familial tendencies, also explore the patient's family history.

Because SLE can affect almost every body system, use a body-systems approach when performing the physical examination. (See *Diagnostic criteria for SLE*, page 28.)

Continued on page 28

Autoimmune Disorders

Diagnostic criteria for SLE

Diagnosing systemic lupus erythematosus (SLE) presents special problems. Symptoms vary greatly from one patient to another and appear in widely unpredictable patterns.

To aid diagnosis of SLE, the American Rheumatism Association has developed a list of 11 classification criteria. Any patient meeting four or more of these criteria simultaneously or sequentially in the absence of other causative factors is considered to have SLE. These criteria include:
- butterfly rash
- discoid rash
- photosensitivity
- oral or nasopharyngeal ulcers, usually painless
- nonerosive arthritis affecting two or more peripheral joints
- serositis, marked by pleuritis or pericarditis
- renal disorder, marked by persistent proteinuria greater than 0.5 g/day (or greater than 3+) or by cellular casts (red blood cell, hemoglobulin, granular, tubular, or mixed)
- neurologic disorder, marked by seizures or psychoses
- hematologic disorder marked by hemolytic anemia with reticulocytosis, leukopenia, lymphopenia, or thrombocytopenia
- immunologic disorder, marked by positive LE cell preparation, or anti-DNA antibody, or anti-Smith antigen or by false-positive serologic test for syphilis for at least 6 months
- abnormal antinuclear antibodies (ANA) titer.

Systemic lupus erythematosus—*continued*

Skin. Rash, a common sign, ranges from erythema to discoid plaques. Typically, it appears on areas exposed to sunlight, such as the scalp, face, and neck. Also look for two uncommon but telltale signs of SLE: butterfly rash (a maculopapular eruption across the nose and cheeks) and erythema of the fingertips or palms. During periods of active disease, you may observe patchy or diffuse alopecia; however, hair usually grows back during remission. Oral and genital ulcers may develop in some patients. (See *Discoid lupus erythematosus* for specifics on another organ-nonspecific disorder.)

Musculoskeletal system. Assess for joint symptoms. Fleeting polyarthralgia or arthritis affects about 90% of patients with the disorder. Almost any joint may be involved in this symmetrical arthritis. Redness, warmth, tenderness, and synovial effusions may occur. Myalgias commonly occur, sometimes including myositis.

SLE arthritis differs from rheumatoid arthritis in its absence of bony erosion and severe deformity. Avascular necrosis of bone, especially of the femoral head, often develops, but this may stem from corticosteroid therapy rather than from SLE.

Cardiovascular system. Pericarditis, usually mild and self-limiting, may be an early sign. Be alert for complaints of mild chest discomfort. Auscultation may reveal a pericardial friction rub. Affected patients may also develop myocarditis or endocarditis.

In active SLE, vasculitis almost invariably develops in small vessels. It most commonly affects the digits and extremities, producing splinter hemorrhages, periungual occlusions, finger pulp, infarctions, and atrophic ulcers. Gastrointestinal vasculitis can cause abdominal pain, diarrhea, hemorrhage, pancreatitis, and cholecystitis. Involvement of small- to medium-sized arteries can produce complications ranging from bowel infarction to cerebrovascular accident.

Raynaud's phenomenon occurs in about 15% of patients with SLE; severe cases can cause gangrene of the digits. Coronary artery disease may develop in patients receiving long-term corticosteroid therapy.

Renal system. Renal involvement may have serious consequences, so frequent assessment is vital. Lupus nephritis affects about 75% of patients, producing hypertension and renal dysfunction, which may progress to renal failure. (See *Classifying lupus nephritis*, page 30.) Symptoms may be mild or may include anuria, depending on the type of lesion and disease activity.

Nervous system. SLE often causes central nervous system (CNS) effects, such as emotional instability, psychosis, depression, migraine headaches, and seizures. Cranial nerve palsies and peripheral neuritis (most commonly the typical "stocking-glove" pattern affecting the hands and feet) also may occur.

Respiratory system. Be alert for dyspnea and pleuritic chest pain. However, keep in mind that restrictive interstitial lung disease, which occurs commonly among SLE patients, usually produces no symptoms and appears only when pulmonary function tests are performed. Rarely, SLE produces pneumonitis.

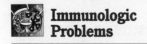

Autoimmune Disorders

Discoid lupus erythematosus

A benign cutaneous disorder, discoid lupus erythematosus (DLE) produces chronic skin eruptions consisting of well-circumscribed red or purple scaling plaques with follicular plugging and central atrophy. It mainly strikes women between ages 20 and 60, with peak incidence at ages 35 to 45.

DLE may be classified as localized (with lesions confined to the face, scalp, and neck) or generalized (with lesions occurring anywhere on the body). These lesions may persist for months or even years. If untreated, they can result in permanent scarring. Although systemic involvement and extracutaneous lesions don't occur in DLE as they do in systemic lupus erythematosus (SLE), DLE progresses to SLE in as many as 15% of patients.

Immunofluorescent testing of skin lesions shows deposits of immunoglobulin and complement at the dermal-epidermal junction. In DLE, this lupus band test is positive only in involved skin; in SLE, the band is present in uninvolved skin as well. Serum immunologic tests usually show normal results, although the erythrocyte sedimentation rate may be elevated in active DLE and some patients may demonstrate positive antinuclear antibody titers.

A patient with DLE should avoid prolonged exposure to sunlight. He also should wear protective clothing and apply a sunscreen with a high skin protection factor before going out in the sun. Drug therapy may involve intralesional injection of triamcinolone acetonide, local application of fluorinated steroid ointment, or administration of systemic antimalarials (such as chloroquine or hydroxychloroquine) or low-dose prednisone.

Gastrointestinal system. Ask about nausea, vomiting, anorexia, or abdominal pain. These can signal such GI disorders as pancreatitis, acute or chronic hepatitis, peritonitis, or GI ulcers.

Eyes. About 25% of patients with SLE develop some form of ocular involvement. Retinal vasculitis, the most common effect, produces white fluffy exudates on the retina, indicating focal nerve fiber degeneration. Scleritis and corneal ulcers also may occur.

Other. Polyserositis, with usually mild pleural, pericardial, and peritoneal effusions, occurs in about one third of patients. About 5% to 10% of patients develop the sicca complex of Sjögren's syndrome, with keratoconjunctivitis sicca (dry eyes, leading to pain, itching, and redness) and xerostomia (dry mouth). Lymph node enlargement, usually nontender, may occur in active SLE. Women often experience irregular or heavy menses.

Diagnostic tests. Various tests help diagnose and monitor SLE. The CBC with differential may show normochromic normocytic anemia in about 80% of patients resulting from bone marrow suppression. It may also show leukopenia and thrombocytopenia. Partial thromboplastin and prothrombin times may be prolonged—the result of circulating anticoagulant antibodies. The serum albumin/globulin ratio may be reversed because of increased immunoglobulins, especially IgG. Erythrocyte sedimentation rate (ESR) often rises, particularly in active stages. Urinalysis may show hematuria, proteinuria, and red and white blood cell casts.

Immunologic tests reveal considerable autoimmune activity. Reduced levels of serum complement C3 and C4, caused by immune complex formation, occur in active disease. Levels of C5 to C9, though, may rise in active disease. Measurement of complement levels may help in managing SLE. A reduced C4 level is the most sensitive indicator of disease activity.

The presence of autoantibodies is the most characteristic abnormal laboratory finding in SLE. Direct immunofluorescence testing for antinuclear antibodies (ANA) usually reveals high titers. In fact, absence of ANA is considered strong evidence against a diagnosis of SLE. (See *Antinuclear antibodies*, page 30.) Anti-DNA antibodies, detected by radioimmunoassay, also characteristically appear in SLE. In fact, one type—anti–double-stranded or "native" DNA antibodies—occurs almost exclusively in SLE. Antierythrocyte antibodies, detected using the direct Coombs' test, also may appear in SLE.

Rheumatoid factor may rise in about one third of patients with SLE, evidenced by a positive latex fixation test. A false-positive serologic test for syphilis occurs in 10% to 20% of patients.

In almost 90% of patients with SLE, tissue immunofluorescence testing identifies IgG and IgM as well as complement deposition in the epidermal-dermal junction of skin that's unaffected by an active lupus rash. In contrast, patients with discoid lupus erythematosus show immunoglobulin and complement deposition only in involved skin. In lupus nephritis, electron microscopy usually reveals irregular or granular immunoglobulin and complement accumulation on the glomerular basement membrane and in the mesangium.

Continued on page 30

Autoimmune Disorders

Classifying lupus nephritis

Lupus nephritis may be classified into four types.

Mesangial glomerulonephritis, a benign form, is marked by cellular proliferation and immune complex deposition in the mesangium.

In *focal glomerulonephritis*, cellular proliferation occurs in less than half of the glomeruli. Immune complexes are deposited in the mesangium and the glomerular capillary subendothelium.

Usually benign, focal glomerulonephritis occasionally progresses to *diffuse proliferative glomerulonephritis*. This type of lupus nephritis is characterized by extensive cellular proliferation in more than half the glomeruli and immune complex deposition, mainly in the subendothelium. It often results in renal failure.

In *membranous glomerulonephritis*, usually associated with renal failure, no glomerular cell changes occur, but the capillary basement membrane thickens. Immune complexes are deposited mainly in subepithelial and intramembranous areas.

Antinuclear antibodies

Autoantibodies directed against components of cell nuclei, antinuclear antibodies (ANA) appear in various autoimmune diseases, particularly systemic lupus erythematosus (SLE). Immunofluorescent staining detects four different patterns of ANA activity.

The *homogenous (diffuse or solid) pattern* occurs in patients with systemic or drug-induced lupus erythematosus. In this pattern, the nucleus shows uniform, diffuse staining.

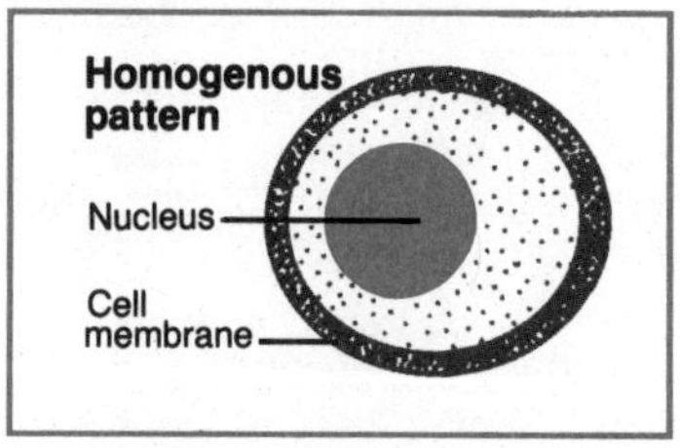

The *peripheral (shaggy or outline) pattern*, characteristic of active SLE, reveals anti–double-stranded DNA antibodies.

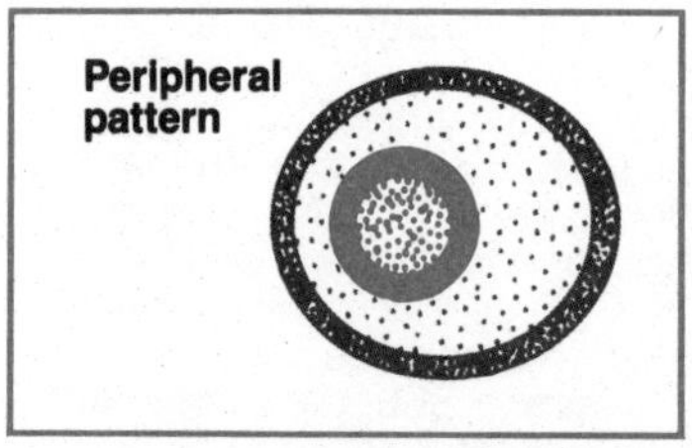

The *speckled pattern* reflects the presence of antibodies directed against non-DNA nuclear constituents. The anti–ENA (extractable nuclear antigen) assay detects antibodies against the Smith (Sm) antigen and ribonucleoprotein (RNP) antigen. Antibodies against the Sm antigen are characteristic of SLE. High anti-RNP antibody titers are the hallmarks of mixed connective tissue disease. This speckled pattern may occur in SLE, rheumatoid arthritis, Sjögren's syndrome, and progressive systemic sclerosis (PSS).

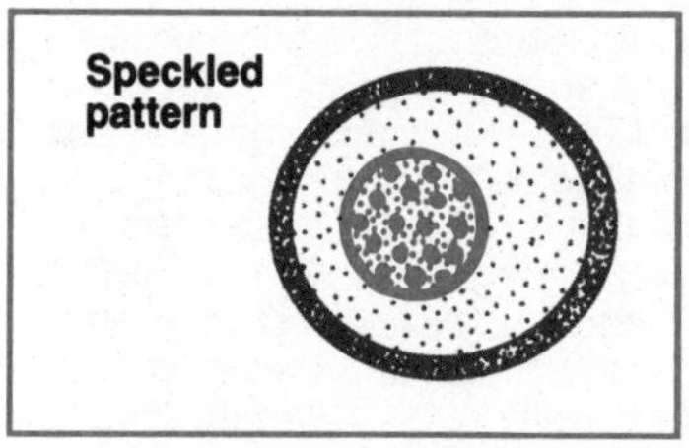

The *nucleolar pattern* shows homogenous staining of the nucleolus. This antigen's pattern is most often associated with PSS or polymyositis and dermatomyositis.

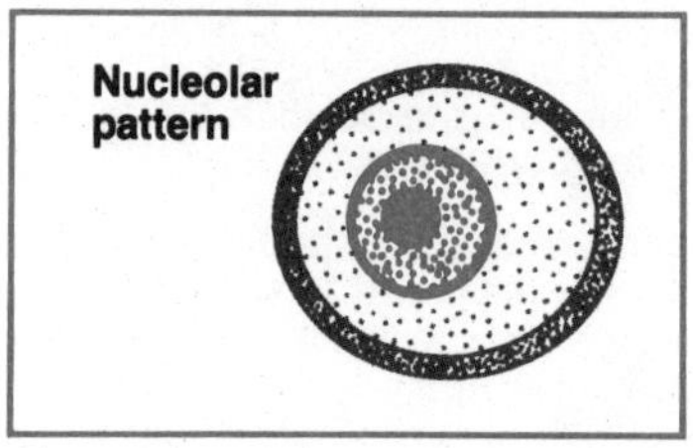

Systemic lupus erythematosus—*continued*

Planning

Before determining your nursing care plan, develop the nursing diagnosis by identifying your patient's problem or potential problem, then relating it to its cause. Possible nursing diagnoses for a patient with SLE include:

- activity intolerance (fatigue); related to disease process
- bowel elimination, alteration in (diarrhea); related to bowel wall inflammation or GI tract vasculitis
- cardiac output, alteration in (decreased); related to pericardial or myocardial inflammation
- thought processes, alteration in (confusion); related to cerebral inflammation
- tissue perfusion, alteration in peripheral (decreased); related to small vessel occlusion by inflammatory process
- urinary elimination, alteration in patterns (decreased); related to renal insufficiency or failure

Autoimmune Disorders

- self-concept, disturbance in body image; related to corticosteroid use
- hopelessness; related to disease prognosis.

The sample nursing care plan on page 32 shows expected outcomes, nursing interventions, and discharge planning for one nursing diagnosis listed above. However, you'll want to tailor each care plan to your patient's needs.

Intervention
Treatment priorities in SLE include relieving symptoms, correcting abnormalities noted on laboratory tests, and preventing organ damage. Specific interventions depend on SLE's severity and stage. They range from general health promotion measures—adequate rest, good nutrition, moderate exercise, and avoidance of sunlight—to such intensive therapies as high-dose immunosuppressants and plasmapheresis. Teaching the patient and his family about prevention and treatment measures also figures prominently in long-term management.

Drug therapy. Drug therapy for SLE patients may include aspirin or other nonsteroidal anti-inflammatory drugs (NSAIDs), antimalarials, corticosteroids, or immunosuppressants. Aspirin or NSAIDs given at 4 g daily or more may relieve arthritic symptoms and fever. However, NSAIDs are contraindicated in patients with compromised renal perfusion or renal insufficiency because they may impair glomerular filtration. (See *Reviewing nonsteroidal anti-inflammatory drugs*, page 33.) Antimalarial drugs, such as hydroxychloroquine and chloroquine, often prove effective in treating skin and mucosal lesions. However, such therapy requires low doses and careful monitoring to prevent retinal damage.

Systemic corticosteroids are usually the drugs of choice for treating severe systemic symptoms and acute exacerbations. High-dose therapy may be indicated in acute fulminant disease, acute lupus nephritis, acute CNS effects, acute autoimmune hemolytic anemia, or thrombocytopenic purpura. Initial high doses may bring rapid improvement; after improvement, the dosage should be tapered gradually and, if possible, the drug eventually discontinued. However, extensive or persistent renal involvement may require continued corticosteroid therapy. Topical corticosteroids, such as flurandrenolide, also can help clear up skin or mucosal lesions.

Keep in mind that long-term corticosteroid use can cause severe adverse reactions. Be sure to monitor the patient carefully and teach him about early signs of such reactions.

Immunosuppressive drugs, such as cyclophosphamide, chlorambucil, methotrexate, and azathioprine, may prove effective if other drugs fail to improve the patient's condition, especially if he has lupus nephritis. However, these drugs can cause severe adverse reactions, requiring extra caution during use.

Plasmapheresis. This procedure—involving mechanical removal of toxins from the blood—may offer temporary benefits during acute episodes, especially for patients with lupus cerebritis or rapidly progressive lupus nephritis. This procedure usually accompanies

Continued on page 32

Autoimmune Disorders

Sample nursing care plan: Systemic lupus erythematosus

Nursing diagnosis	Expected outcomes
Activity intolerance (fatigue); related to the disease process	The patient will: • explain the relationship between fatigue and his disease. • describe the psychological and physiologic factors that may cause fatigue and be able to differentiate between them. • identify measures to prevent or minimize fatigue. • employ these measures himself, and request that caregivers do so as well. • tolerate selected activities without becoming fatigued.
Nursing interventions	**Discharge planning**
• Teach the patient and his family about the relationship between fatigue and systemic lupus erythematosus. Explain that increased fatigue may herald exacerbations. • Explain physiologic and psychological factors affecting the severity and duration of fatigue. Physiologic factors include anemia from chronic disease, energy consumption by cells involved in the immune response, poor nutrition, drug effects, muscle atrophy, and sleep disruption from persistent discomfort. Psychological factors include stress, anxiety, pain, emotional well-being, and the side effects of drug therapy. • Plan the patient's care schedule to allow for uninterrupted nighttime sleep and frequent rest periods throughout the day. • Provide pain management measures and assess their effectiveness. • Use stress-reduction techniques and help the patient develop his own coping strategies. • Encourage the patient to maintain adequate nutritional intake. • Encourage physical activity, as appropriate, to prevent or minimize muscle atrophy.	• Teach the patient energy-conserving measures, including planning a 30- to 45-minute rest period each morning and each afternoon (longer periods may worsen joint stiffness); setting priorities on goals to avoid overexertion or stress; pacing activities to take advantage of energetic periods; using proper body mechanics and assistive devices to conserve energy; sitting rather than standing when possible; maintaining good posture; and asking family members or others for help when necessary. • Include family members in your teaching, if appropriate. Make sure they understand that fatigue is a sign of disease and not a psychological problem. • As appropriate, refer the patient for occupational or vocational counseling. • Teach pain management techniques. • Explain stress-reduction techniques. • Review the patient's understanding of the disease and its treatment; reinforce the care plan. • Arrange for appropriate follow-up care. • Advise the patient when to seek medical attention.

Systemic lupus erythematosus—*continued*

corticosteroid and cyclophosphamide therapy. (See *Plasmapheresis*, page 34.)

Supportive care. Supportive measures depend on the patient's symptoms and the disease severity. At times, these measures focus on treating specific organ involvement, such as hypertension in kidney failure.

Prevention and early treatment of infection remains a prime concern because both the disease and its treatment are immunosuppressive. As a result, the patient and his caregivers must be alert for signs of infection—signs that are often masked in immunosuppressed patients.

Other supportive measures include:
• ensuring proper nutrition. Encourage the patient to eat a balanced diet and adhere to any dietary restrictions.
• instructing him to get adequate rest and to pace his work and other activities to avoid overexertion.

Autoimmune Disorders

Reviewing nonsteroidal anti-inflammatory drugs

Drugs	Adverse reactions	Nursing considerations
Salicylates • acetylsalicylic acid • magnesium salicylate • salsalate • diflunisal	Constipation, GI irritation, hearing loss, prolonged bleeding time, tinnitus	• Administer with a full glass of water, with meals, or with an antacid to minimize GI irritation.
Proprionic acid derivatives • ibuprofen • naproxen • fenoprofen • carprofen	Diarrhea, dizziness, dyspepsia, GI irritation, headache, heartburn, nausea, rash, renal failure, renal toxicity (especially if patient has impaired renal function), vomiting	• For optimum absorption, administer at least 30 minutes before or at least 2 hours after meals. • Tell patient to promptly report any adverse reactions.
Indomethacin-related drugs • indomethacin • tolmetin	Congestive heart failure; edema; GI irritation, ulceration, or bleeding; headache; nephritis; prolonged bleeding time	• Administer with food to minimize GI irritation. • Tell patient to restrict sodium intake while taking drug. • Instruct patient to promptly report any signs of bleeding.
Fenamates • mefenamic acid • meclofenamate	Bone marrow hypoplasia, diarrhea, dyspepsia, edema, nausea, rash, vomiting	• Instruct patient to restrict sodium intake while taking drug.
Oxicams • piroxicam	Anemia, constipation, diarrhea, dizziness, dyspepsia, edema, headache, nausea, pruritus, rash, tinnitus	• Tell patient to promptly report any adverse reactions.
Pyrazolones • phenylbutazone • oxyphenbutazone	Bone marrow suppression, dizziness, dyspepsia, edema, liver damage, peptic ulcer, rash	• Instruct the patient to promptly report any signs of bleeding, easy bruising, or mouth sores. • Drug shouldn't be used for longer than 7 days if no response because of potentially severe toxic effects.

• encouraging the photosensitive patient to reduce his exposure to sunlight, to wear protective clothing, and to use a sunscreen that contains para-aminobenzoic acid when outdoors. In severe photosensitivity, urge the patient to avoid excessive exposure to indoor fluorescent lights.
• teaching the patient and his family, if appropriate, about SLE, including how to recognize early signs of flare-ups and how to prevent or minimize symptoms and complications.
• providing emotional support. Loss of independence and feeling out of control are major problems for many SLE patients. Body image changes caused by the disease and its treatment can be disturbing. And the fatigue, discomfort, and inconveniences of SLE may add to the patient's emotional distress.
• referring the patient and his family to a local SLE support group or providing them with local addresses for the National Lupus Erythematosus Foundation and the Arthritis Foundation.

Evaluation

Base your evaluation on the expected outcomes listed on the nursing care plan. To determine if the patient has improved, ask yourself the following questions:
• Is the patient able to discuss the relationship between fatigue and disease activity?
• Does he know what factors predispose him to fatigue?
• Is he aware of methods to lessen or prevent fatigue?
• Does he use these methods?
• Is the patient better able to tolerate selected activities?

Continued on page 35

Autoimmune Disorders

Plasmapheresis

Used to treat patients with systemic lupus erythematosus, Guillain-Barré syndrome, multiple sclerosis, and myasthenia gravis, plasmapheresis (also known as therapeutic plasma exchange, or TPE) mechanically removes such unwanted substances as toxins, metabolic wastes, and plasma constituents implicated in disease (such as immune complexes and circulating autoantibodies).

In this treatment, blood removed from the patient flows into a cell separator, which divides it into plasma and formed elements. The plasma is collected for disposal, and the formed elements are mixed with plasma replacement solution and returned to the patient.

During plasmapheresis, monitor the patient closely for signs and symptoms of potential complications, which include allergic reaction, citrate-induced hypocalcemia, clotting problems, fluid imbalance, hemorrhage caused by anticoagulant administration, infection from replacement fluids, and hemolysis. The machine's safety features help ensure maximum plasma flow and optimum separation; they also help prevent complications. The diagram below shows how a typical plasmapheresis system works.

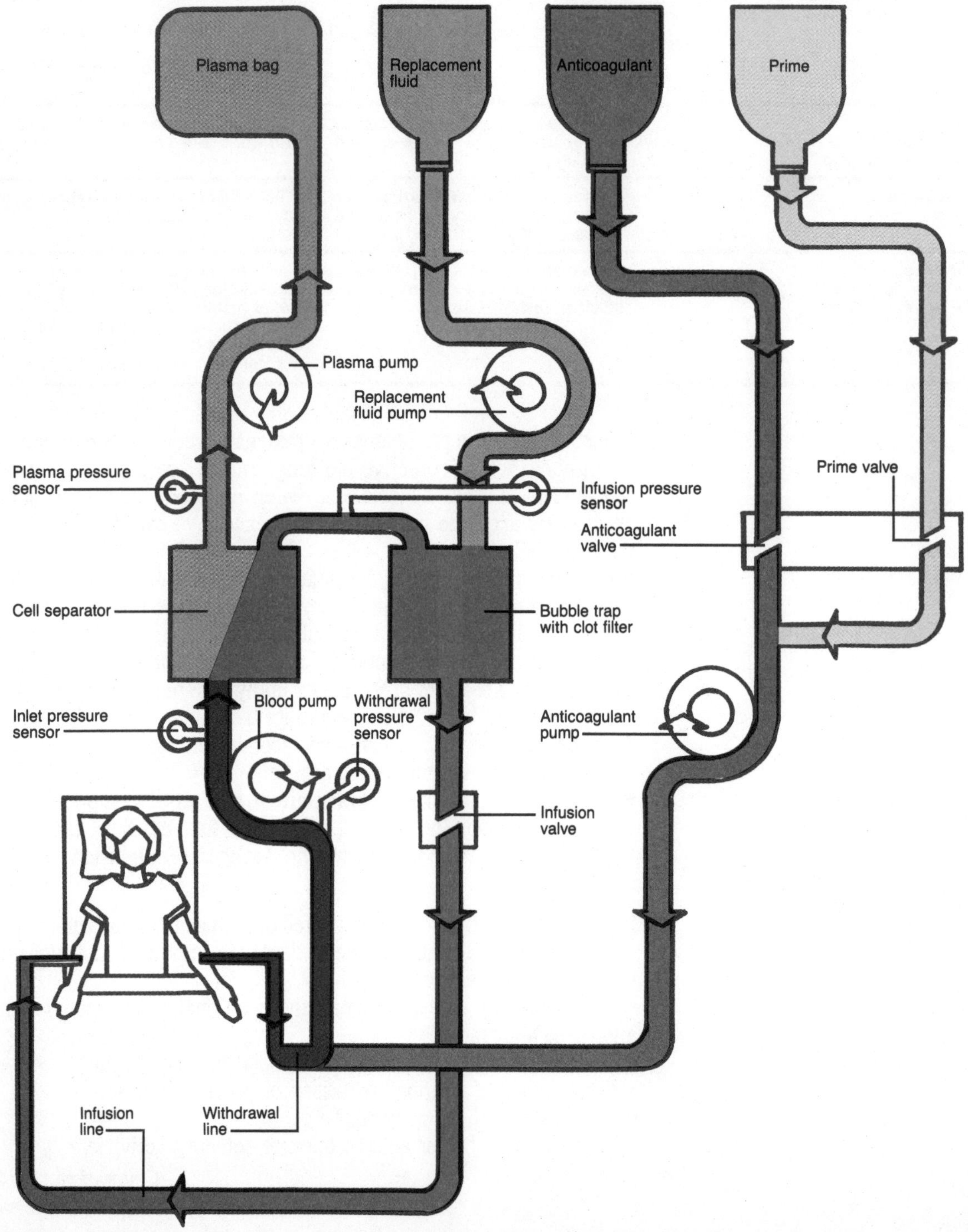

Autoimmune Disorders

Systemic lupus erythematosus—*continued*

The answers to these questions will help you evaluate your patient's status and the effectiveness of the care plan. Keep in mind that these questions stem from the sample nursing care plan on page 32; your specific questions may differ.

Other organ-nonspecific autoimmune disorders

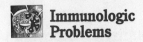

Besides SLE, other systemic autoimmune disorders include rheumatoid arthritis, Sjögren's syndrome, progressive systemic sclerosis, Goodpasture's syndrome, polymyositis, dermatomyositis, and serum sickness.

Specific musculoskeletal-related pathogenesis, signs and symptoms, and treatment of rheumatoid arthritis and related disorders appear in detail in the NURSEREVIEW section on "Musculoskeletal Problems." This section focuses on the disorders' autoimmune aspects.

Rheumatoid arthritis
A chronic, recurrent inflammatory disorder of connective tissue, rheumatoid arthritis (RA) primarily affects bones, tendons, cartilage, ligaments, and the intima of blood vessels. RA usually develops insidiously, with symptoms beginning in the small joints of the hands and feet before progressing gradually to such large joints as the knees, elbows, and shoulders. Joint involvement characteristically occurs symmetrically. Effects range from mild discomfort to severe, destructive arthritis. In some patients, RA may attack connective tissue in other organs, such as the spleen, lungs, and eyes. The disease strikes women three times more often than men. (See *Diagnostic criteria for rheumatoid arthritis*, page 36.)

Although the cause of RA remains unknown, evidence suggests an immune or autoimmune process. Currently, an antigen is thought to stimulate an immune response marked by abnormal IgG, which leads to production of rheumatoid factor (RF)—an antibody to IgG or IgM—and subsequent RA development. Although researchers haven't identified the antigen, they believe that genetic and environmental factors (such as viruses) play important roles. RA patients display increased HLA-D4 and HLA-DR4; perhaps these and other genetic determinants impart susceptibility to environmental factors.

The major immunologic features of RA include:
- RF in blood and synovial fluid (7S and 19S IgM and 7S IgG)
- reduced complement in synovial fluid. (See *Autoimmune-related rheumatic disorders*, page 36.)

Assessment. Initial assessment focuses on the health history. The patient's chief complaint will probably be joint pain. He may also report fatigue, generalized muscle stiffness and aching, weakness, anorexia, and weight loss. Pain and stiffness may be particularly severe when the patient first rises in the morning; symptoms often subside somewhat during the day.

Be sure to ask about the duration of morning stiffness. A patient with untreated RA may experience stiffness for up to 6 hours after

Continued on page 36

Autoimmune Disorders

Diagnostic criteria for rheumatoid arthritis

To aid diagnosis of rheumatoid arthritis (RA), the American Rheumatism Society has established criteria. For a diagnosis of classic RA, the patient must meet at least seven of these criteria; for definite RA, five; and for probable RA, three. The first five criteria listed below must persist for at least 6 weeks to qualify as diagnostic. Qualifying criteria include:
- morning stiffness
- pain on motion or tenderness in at least one joint
- swelling (soft tissue or fluid) of at least one joint
- swelling of at least one other joint
- symmetrical joint swelling (same joint, both left and right)
- subcutaneous nodules
- X-ray changes typical of RA
- positive serum test for rheumatoid factors
- poor mucin clotting of synovial fluid
- characteristic histologic changes in synovium
- characteristic histologic changes in rheumatoid nodules.

Autoimmune-related rheumatic disorders

Various rheumatic disorders may involve autoimmune mechanisms. Besides rheumatoid arthritis, the list includes:
- Ankylosing spondylitis
- Behçet's disease
- Giant cell arteritis
- Henoch-Schönlein purpura
- Hypersensitivity angiitis
- Juvenile arthritis
- Polyarteritis nodosa
- Reiter's syndrome
- Takayasu's arteritis
- Wegener's granulomatosis

Other organ-nonspecific disorders—*continued*

awakening, whereas one with controlled disease may report morning stiffness lasting 30 minutes or less. Because RA seems to have a genetic predisposition, ask the patient if any other family member has had RA or any of its symptoms.

During the physical examination, assess each joint for warmth, pain, and nodules. Observe for such signs of inflammation as redness, swelling, contractures, and limited range of motion. Take the patient's "joint count" by adding the number of painful joints; the higher the number, the more active the disease. Also assess surrounding muscle and soft tissue. Look for soft tissue swelling and muscle atrophy, and test muscle strength in affected limbs.

Diagnostic tests. Several tests aid diagnosis. The RF test shows positive results (a titer of 1:80 or higher) in 70% to 80% of patients with RA; RF titers usually correlate with disease severity. However, because RF appears in 1% to 5% of patients who don't have RA, positive RF results alone will not confirm a diagnosis of RA.

ESR nearly always rises during active disease. It may be normal early in the disease, but C-reactive protein levels will rise in acute stages.

Interventions. For most patients, treatment includes drug therapy and supportive measures. It aims to minimize inflammation, thereby avoiding joint and connective tissue damage.

Drug therapy. Aspirin and other NSAIDs are often prescribed to suppress the inflammatory or immune response.

Corticosteroids, antimalarials, gold salts, and penicillamine may help control inflammation, thus reducing symptoms and possibly slowing disease progress. Although just how these drugs exert their beneficial effects remains unclear, they apparently act as immunosuppressive agents, altering the function of cells involved in rheumatoid inflammation.

Immunosuppressive agents, such as azathioprine, cyclophosphamide, and methotrexate, also may provide benefits in severe RA. However, because of the risks involved in immunosuppressive therapy, these drugs usually are reserved for patients unresponsive to other treatments. Guanethidine, under investigation for RA treatment, may be given as a single I.V. injection to relieve joint pain.

Supportive care. Encourage therapeutic exercises to help maintain muscle strength and joint range of motion. Urge the patient to get adequate sleep, take rest periods between activities, and learn principles of joint protection. Advise heat treatments to help ease muscle spasm, stiffness, and pain. Teach the patient and his caregivers about the chronic, recurrent nature of RA and what they can do to minimize its effects.

Surgery. Such techniques as arthroplasty or joint replacement may be needed to improve joint motion, correct deformity, and help relieve pain.

Autoimmune Disorders

Carprofen: A new NSAID

Recently approved by the Food and Drug Administration, carprofen (Rimadyl) is a member of the proprionic acid class of nonsteroidal anti-inflammatory drugs (NSAIDs), which includes ibuprofen and naproxen. Carprofen also possesses analgesic and antipyretic activity.

The drug can be used to treat rheumatoid arthritis, osteoarthritis, ankylosing spondylitis, tendinitis and bursitis, dental and post-traumatic pain, and gout. Dosage ranges from 150 to 600 mg/day P.O., in two or three divided doses.

Rapidly and extensively absorbed after administration, carprofen reaches peak concentrations in 1 to 3 hours (perhaps slightly longer in elderly patients). Food ingestion causes slightly reduced absorption rate and peak concentration. The drug is metabolized in the liver and excreted mainly in the urine.

Adverse effects include acute renal failure, abdominal pain, dyspepsia, dysuria, eczema, heartburn, hematuria, nausea, nephritis, photosensitivity, proteinuria, rash, urinary frequency, and urticaria.

Sjögren's syndrome

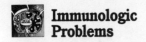

A chronic inflammatory disorder characterized by diminished lacrimal and salivary secretions, Sjögren's syndrome may occur alone or with other autoimmune disorders, such as RA or SLE. It strikes nine times more women than men. Its cause isn't known, but genetic factors (including a strong association with the histocompatibility antigens HLA-B8 and HLA-DR3) and immunologic processes (specifically, excessive B-cell and depressed T-cell activity) are suspected.

Immunologic features of Sjögren's syndrome include:

- hypergammaglobulinemia
- ANA
- RF
- autoantibodies to salivary duct and other antigens
- elevated salivary beta$_2$-microglobulin level
- lymphocyte and plasma cell infiltration in involved tissue.

Assessment. Primary features include keratoconjunctivitis sicca and xerostomia. Assessment also may reveal enlarged salivary glands; an ulcerated, fissured (geographic) tongue; and dry, erythematous oral mucosa. The patient may complain of nasal, throat, and vaginal dryness. In some patients, Raynaud's phenomenon and lymphadenopathy may occur.

Diagnostic tests. These may include Schirmer's tear test to detect decreased lacrimal secretions and biopsy of minor salivary glands to confirm lymphocyte infiltration.

Other common test findings include an elevated ESR (in more than 90% of patients), hypergammaglobulinemia (in 50%), leukopenia (in 30%), and normochromic anemia (in about 25%).

Interventions. Because no known cure exists for Sjögren's syndrome, treatment focuses on symptomatic relief. Measures commonly include use of methylcellulose artificial tears to relieve dry eyes and artificial saliva or lozenges to relieve dry mouth. A bedroom humidifier may help relieve symptoms at night. NSAIDs may help relieve arthritic symptoms. Corticosteroids, immunosuppressants, or cytotoxic drugs may be used to treat severe systemic manifestations.

To help minimize symptoms, encourage the patient to maintain good oral hygiene, with regular use of fluoride-containing toothpaste and mouthwash and regular dental examinations. Also advise the patient that sipping water or chewing sugarless gum or candy can help relieve dry mouth.

Progressive systemic sclerosis

A chronic disease of unknown etiology, progressive systemic sclerosis (PSS), also known as scleroderma, produces diffuse fibrosis in skin and internal organs accompanied by proliferative arterial occlusions. PSS occurs in all races and affects women three times more often than men. It typically appears between ages 20 and 30 and follows a slowly progressive course leading to chronic disability. However, it may progress rapidly to death in some patients.

Continued on page 38

Autoimmune Disorders

Mixed connective tissue disease

Consisting of features of progressive systemic sclerosis, systemic lupus erythematosus, and polymyositis and dermatomyositis, mixed connective tissue disease (MCTD) produces such effects as arthritis, Raynaud's phenomenon, sclerodactyly, muscle tenderness and weakness, interstitial lung disease, and a rash resembling that seen in either SLE or dermatomyositis. Affected patients also exhibit high speckled-pattern antinuclear antibody titers and antibody to the ribonuclease-sensitive component of extractable nuclear antigen. Renal involvement rarely occurs. Patients usually benefit from corticosteroids in moderate doses.

Other organ-nonspecific disorders—*continued*

Although the etiology of PSS is unclear, the disorder's association with Sjögren's syndrome and sometimes thyroiditis, along with characteristic immunologic features (ANA, RF, polyclonal hypergammaglobulinemia), suggests an autoimmune dysfunction. However, unlike other autoimmune disorders, PSS is characterized by absent or slight cellular infiltration in all organs but the synovium, where infiltration of lymphocytes and plasma cells is often massive.

Assessment. In more than half of affected patients, PSS begins with Raynaud's phenomenon. When cutaneous involvement appears, effects typically progress in three phases. In the *edematous phase*, symmetrical nonpitting edema develops in the hands and—rarely—the feet and may progress to the arms, upper chest, abdomen, back, and face. In the *sclerotic phase*, skin becomes tight, smooth, and waxy; skin folds and wrinkles disappear. These effects occur mainly in the hands, accompanied by painful slow-healing fingertip ulcers. The patient's face takes on a stretched, masklike appearance, her lips thin, and her nose becomes "pinched." Pigment changes and telangiectasias also may appear during this phase. The skin may stabilize for a time at this phase, then may either return to normal or may progress to the final *atrophic phase*.

Besides experiencing skin changes, the patient may experience joint pain, swelling, and stiffness. Muscle wasting and inflammatory myopathy may also develop. GI involvement produces dysphagia, gastroesophageal reflux, and heartburn. The patient may also complain of abdominal cramps, bloating, and alternating diarrhea and constipation. Slowed GI motility commonly occurs. Lung fibrosis with dyspnea on exertion is also common, as is cor pulmonale. Renal involvement, although rare, may prove life-threatening.

Some PSS patients develop the CREST syndrome: calcinosis, Raynaud's phenomenon, esophageal dysfunction, sclerodactyly, and telangiectasia. This syndrome typically evolves slowly, with gradually worsening skin and visceral involvement.

Other PSS patients may have features of such connective tissue disorders as RA, SLE, or polymyositis and dermatomyositis—a situation sometimes classified as mixed connective tissue disease. (See *Mixed connective tissue disease*.)

Diagnostic tests. Results pointing to a diagnosis of PSS include normochromic normocytic anemia, elevated ESR, polyclonal hypergammaglobulinemia, and a speckled or nucleolar ANA pattern.

Interventions. No cure exists for PSS. Treatment focuses on symptomatic relief, preservation of body functions, and minimizing complications. Vasodilating agents, particularly calcium channel blockers, may relieve severe Raynaud's phenomenon. Sympathectomy has provided only transient relief of vascular symptoms. Penicillamine, on the other hand, may help slow progression of visceral disease and also is often effective in relieving cutaneous manifestations. Colchicine may provide limited cutaneous relief. Although

Autoimmune Disorders

Autoimmune-related glomerulonephritis

About half of all cases of end-stage renal failure can be attributed to immunologically induced glomerulonephritis. Both soluble (circulating) and insoluble (fixed) antigens may be involved, and the immune complexes formed can attack the glomerulus directly or release products that cause glomerular damage.

Two types of autoimmune-related glomerulonephritis are antiglomerular basement membrane (GBM) antibody-induced glomerulonephritis and immune complex glomerulonephritis. Immunologic features of the anti-GBM antibody-induced type include linear deposition of immunoglobulin and possibly complement along the GBM, and anti-GBM antibodies detectable in serum by radioimmunoassay or, less often, by indirect immunofluorescence. In immune complex glomerulonephritis, granular deposition of immunoglobulins and complement occurs in the glomeruli. In some cases, circulating immune complexes may be detected. Types of immune complex glomerulonephritis include proliferative, membranous, membroproliferative, and end-stage (chronic) glomerulonephritis.

Besides supportive care, treatment for these disorders may include immunosuppressive therapy, corticosteroid therapy, or both. For anti-GBM antibody-induced glomerulonephritis, it may include plasmapheresis. Kidney transplantation may prove beneficial for patients with immune complex glomerulonephritis, but only after nephrogenic immune complex production has fallen to minimal or undetectable levels. Recurrence after transplantation has been reported in some patients.

corticosteroids don't arrest the visceral progression of PSS, they may help relieve symptoms in patients with myositis or mixed connective tissue disease. Skin lubricants can relieve dryness and cracking.

Aspirin and other NSAIDs usually can control arthritic symptoms. Captopril may prove useful in treating associated renal disease, although hypertensive crisis associated with severe renal involvement may prove difficult to control even with the most potent antihypertensives. Advise the patient to avoid exposure to cold, to wear gloves to protect his hands, and to avoid tobacco.

Goodpasture's syndrome

Characterized by pulmonary hemorrhage and glomerulonephritis, this syndrome apparently results from circulating anti-glomerular basement membrane (anti-GBM) antibodies and linear deposition of immunoglobulin and complement in alveolar and glomerular basement membranes (see *Autoimmune-related glomerulonephritis*). This potentially fatal syndrome most commonly strikes young men. Although the etiology remains unclear, the syndrome is sometimes preceded by a viral infection or inhalation of volatile hydrocarbons.

Assessment. Primary findings include:
- pulmonary hemorrhage, at times with hemoptysis, dyspnea, and coughing
- slight or gross hematuria.

The chest X-ray may show diffuse hilar infiltrates. Typically, blood urea nitrogen and serum creatinine levels rise, and creatinine clearance declines. Urinalysis may reveal proteinuria.

Immunofluorescence testing of renal or pulmonary biopsy tissue shows linear deposition of antibodies along the glomerular basement membrane or alveolar septa. The presence of anti-GBM antibodies in serum aids in the diagnosis.

Interventions. Timely and aggressive treatment is crucial in halting progression to potentially fatal renal failure or severe pulmonary hemorrhage. Initial measures include high-dose parenteral corticosteroids along with cytotoxic agents. Plasmapheresis may also be used to remove circulating anti-GBM antibodies from the blood. Patients with renal failure may benefit from dialysis; kidney transplantation may take place after anti-GBM antibodies can no longer be detected. Supportive measures include oxygenation and mechanical ventilation, as needed.

Polymyositis and dermatomyositis

In these acute or chronic inflammatory diseases, inflammation causes symmetrical weakness, mainly involving the proximal muscles. Immunologic features include:
- presence of ANA to polymyositis antigen
- infiltration of lymphocytes and plasma into involved muscle
- production of cytotoxic lymphokine by lymphocytes incubated with autologous muscle
- presence of focal complement and immunoglobulin (IgG and IgM) depositions in vessel walls of involved tissue.

Continued on page 40

Autoimmune Disorders

Other organ-nonspecific disorders—*continued*

Assessment. Typical findings include a history of slowly progressive weakness in the proximal muscles of the arms and legs. The patient may report difficulty getting out of chairs, climbing stairs, or performing other activities of daily living. He also may experience dysphagia from pharyngeal muscle involvement.

The patient with dermatomyositis will also have skin involvement. It appears as a subtle heliotropic rash, affecting only the eyelids and knuckles or possibly covering large body areas.

Diagnostic tests. In polymyositis and dermatomyositis, tests typically show elevated serum creatine phosphokinase and SGOT levels. Electromyography reveals polyphasic short-duration potentials and other characteristic abnormalities.

Interventions. Corticosteroids, such as prednisone, are the treatment of choice. If the patient doesn't respond to corticosteroids, such immunosuppressants as methotrexate or azathioprine may be administered.

Serum sickness
Considered the prototypical immune complex disorder, serum sickness involves an adverse immunologic reaction to a foreign antigen (usually a heterologous protein). It may occur after administration of various heterologous antitoxins (including those for rabies, diphtheria, snake venom, and *Clostridia*) or certain drugs, such as penicillin or sulfonamides. The initial immune response results in antigen excess, leading to the formation of soluble antigen-antibody complexes. These complexes diffuse into involved tissues, activating complement and initiating the inflammatory response that causes the disorder. Rising antibody titers result in formation of insoluble complexes that are rapidly cleared by the mononuclear phagocyte system.

Assessment. Signs of serum sickness usually develop 7 to 15 days after exposure to the offending antigen. Initial signs include fever, muscle pain and weakness, joint pain and stiffness, urticaria, lymphadenopathy, and splenomegaly. Arthritic effects may involve both large and small joints, and include pain, swelling, and effusions; they usually don't include warmth and redness. Diagnostic tests show leukocytosis, hematuria, proteinuria, and decreased complement levels.

Interventions. Serum sickness usually is self-limiting, with no serious complications. Treatment may include epinephrine and antihistamines for urticaria and salicylates for arthritic symptoms. In severe disease, corticosteroids may be used briefly.

Organ-specific autoimmune disorders

These disorders occur when antigens confined to one organ trigger abnormal autoimmune responses. The following chart lists selected organ-specific autoimmune disorders.

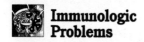

Autoimmune Disorders

Organ-specific autoimmune disorders

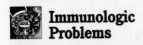

Disorder	Immunologic features and test findings	Signs and symptoms	Interventions
CARDIAC DISORDERS			
Acute rheumatic fever	• Follows group A streptococcal pharyngitis • Genetic predisposition • Formation of antibodies to streptococcal cellular and extracellular antigens • Presence of cross-reactive antibodies that bind to various host tissues • Presence of lymphocytes that are cytotoxic to cardiac tissue • Elevated white blood cell (WBC) count, erythrocyte sedimentation rate (ESR), C-reactive protein level • Positive group A streptococcal throat culture • Prolonged PR interval on EKG • Increased antistreptolysin O or other streptococcal antibody	• Episode of pharyngitis about 2 to 3 weeks before onset of acute rheumatic symptoms • Arthritis (pain, redness, swelling, and warmth of affected joints) • Cardiac inflammation • Purposeless movements of voluntary muscles, aggravated by stress and alleviated during sleep or rest (Sydenham's chorea) • Circular erythematous rash, commonly on trunk and proximal parts of the limbs • Fever, periumbilical pain	• Antibiotics (usually penicillin or erythromycin) • Bedrest • Symptomatic treatment, such as salicylates for arthritic symptoms
Postcardiac injury syndrome (Dressler's syndrome, postmyocardial infarction syndrome, postpericardiotomy syndrome)	• Elevated levels of antibodies to viral agents • Circulating antibodies to cardiac tissue • Circulating lymphocytes sensitized to mitochondrial extracts of cardiac tissue • Increased WBC count and ESR, positive test for circulating anti-cardiac antibodies (if available)	• Fever after first week following surgery, trauma, or myocardial infarction • Pericarditis (pericardial friction rub, chest pain) • Pleural effusion	• Aspirin for pain • Corticosteroids in severe cases • Pericardiocentesis if cardiac tamponade develops
DERMATOLOGIC DISORDERS			
Bullous pemphigoid	• Separation of epidermis from dermis at lamina lucida • Benign, chronic, self-limiting course • Immunoglobulin and complement deposition on skin's basement membrane • Serum anti-skin basement membrane antibody (present in 80% of patients) • Passive in vivo transfer of the disease with human pemphigoid antibody • Neutrophil and eosinophil chemotactic factors in blister fluid	• Commonly affects elderly patients • Tense, subepidermal, difficult-to-rupture bullae in flexor areas (inguinal, axillae, sides of neck) • Severe pruritus	• Corticosteroid therapy, sometimes combined with azathioprine or methotrexate, usually for 4 to 6 months • Good skin hygiene
Pemphigus vulgaris	• Immunoglobin and complement deposition in squamous intracellular spaces • May resemble burn injury • If untreated, will progress to death by fluid and electrolyte loss and sepsis • Serum antibody directed against intercellular substance of stratified squamous epithelium • Pemphigus IgG promoting epidermal cell detachment in vitro • Increased incidence of HLA-Dw4	• Thin, flaccid bullae within the epidermis (intraepidermal blister), especially on the trunk and scalp, but with no characteristic distribution pattern • Ruptured bullae extend in size • Skin easily denuded by shearing force • Oral and nasal mucosal involvement with extensive oral erosion	• Corticosteroids combined with immunosuppressants—such as azathioprine, methotrexate, or cyclophosphamide—until remission occurs • I.M. gold salts if immunosuppressants and corticosteroids fail • Plasmapheresis if above treatments fail • Fluid, electrolyte, and nutritional support • Careful monitoring for complications—GI bleeding, osteoporosis, and diabetes—resulting from therapy.

Continued on page 42

Autoimmune Disorders

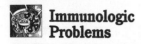

Organ-specific autoimmune disorders—*continued*

Disorder	Immunologic features and test findings	Signs and symptoms	Interventions
ENDOCRINE DISORDERS			
Addison's disease (Idiopathic adrenocortical insufficiency)	• Autoantibodies to adrenal microsomes • Lymphocytic and monocytic infiltration of adrenal glands • Other autoimmune autoantibodies (to gastric parietal cells, thyroglobulin, and intrinsic factor) • Low serum and urine cortisol levels	• Postural hypotension, weight loss, anorexia, weakness, and hyperpigmented skin folds • Other autoimmune diseases, such as diabetes mellitus, ovarian failure, and pernicious anemia	• Replacement of glucocorticoids and mineralocorticoids • Symptomatic and supportive care as needed
Chronic thyroiditis (Hashimoto's thyroiditis)	• Thyroid function tests elevated, depressed, or normal • Autoantibodies to thyroglobulin or thyroid microsomes, or both • Decreased thyroid hormone levels and radioactive iodine uptake; elevated serum thyroid-stimulating hormone and serum cholesterol levels • Self-limited or responsive to thyroid hormone treatment	• Diffusely enlarged thyroid, producing goiter usually firm to hard, only rarely tender, and smooth or scalloped without distinct nodules • Possible severe neck pain radiating to the head • Diminished thyroid function in later stages, suggesting failure of epithelial cell regeneration • Dry skin; coarse, brittle hair; possible myxedema • Low basal metabolic rate	• Administration of thyroid hormone (synthetic thyroxine) • Corticosteroids or immunosuppressive drugs to relieve inflammation • Supportive and symptomatic care • Surgery or radioactive iodine usually not recommended
Diabetes mellitus (type I)	• Circulating antibodies against islet cells • Infiltration of beta cells by lymphocytes, primarily T-suppressor cells but also T-helper cells and natural killer cells • Abnormal deposition of IgG and complement • Both humoral and cell-mediated autoimmune phenomena • Expression of selective aberrant HLA-DR • Possible link to viral infection	• Polyuria • Polydipsia • Polyphagia • Weight loss • Fatigue	• Insulin • Dietary changes • Exercise • Supportive and symptomatic care
Hyperthyroidism	• History of Graves' disease • Autoantibodies directed to thyroid cell surface receptors for thyrotropin or thyroid-stimulating hormone (TSH) • Thyrotropin receptor antibodies that either mimic the stimulatory action of TSH or block TSH binding • Autoantibodies to thyroglobulin or thyroid microsomes, identified by a combination of hemagglutination and immunofluorescence tests • Elevated serum levels of thyroxine and triiodothyronine • Increased uptake of radioactive iodine by the thyroid	• Restlessness, heat intolerance, weight loss, and palpitations • Smooth, warm, moist skin resulting from vasodilation and excessive sweating • Diffuse goiter • Tachycardia, widened pulse pressure, and elevated systolic pressure • Fine tremor of the hands and proximal muscle weakness • Exophthalmos	• Thyroidectomy, administration of radioactive iodine, or antithyroid drugs and adjunctive use of iodine or adrenergic blocking agents • Immunosuppressants rarely necessary; restoration of normal hormone balance appears to decrease inflammation and arrest disease

Autoimmune Disorders

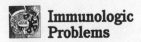

Organ-specific autoimmune disorders—*continued*

Disorder	Immunologic features and test findings	Signs and symptoms	Interventions
GASTROINTESTINAL DISORDERS			
Chronic active hepatitis	• Autoantibodies to liver membrane, smooth muscle, and nuclear antigens • Genetic association with HLA-B8 and HLA-Dw3 • Defect in nonspecific immunoregulation associated with polyclonal hypergammaglobulinemia • Elevated serum bilirubin and aminotransferase levels • Normal or minimally elevated alkaline phosphatase levels • Low serum albumin level and prolonged prothrombin time • Elevated serum IgG, anti-DNA, and antinuclear antibodies	• Usually insidious onset over period of several weeks to months • Chronic hepatic inflammation continuing without improvement for longer than 6 months • Fatigue • Persistent or recurrent jaundice • Malaise for several months before jaundice appears • Anorexia • Recurrent, worsening symptoms suggest acute hepatitis • Complications of cirrhosis (ascites, bleeding esophageal varices, encephalopathy, coagulopathy, hypersplenism)	• Supportive care with adequate rest; return to tolerated activity when remission occurs • Corticosteroids in moderate or low doses, sometimes combined with azathioprine • Continued drug therapy for at least 6 to 12 months, possibly for life if relapse occurs on withdrawal • High-dose corticosteroid therapy for patients unresponsive to other therapy
Inflammatory bowel disease (Crohn's disease, ulcerative colitis)	• Increased numbers of lymphocytes, plasma cells, and monocytes in the mucosa and, in Crohn's disease, the submucosa • Granulomatous response in intestinal lesions and regional lymph nodes in Crohn's disease • Presence of circulating antibodies to cytoplasmic lipopolysaccharides of epithelial cells in colon • Circulating lymphocytotoxic antibodies • Low serum protein levels, serum electrolyte abnormalities • Elevated ESR	• Mild to severe diarrhea; dehydration and electrolyte imbalances in severe diarrhea • Bloody stools • Lower abdominal pain • Fever • Bowel perforation (more common in ulcerative colitis) • Fistula formation between portions of the bowel itself or communicating with skin (perianal), vagina, or bladder (more common in Crohn's disease) • Malabsorption syndrome with malnutrition when small bowel is involved • Oral ulcers in Crohn's disease • Extraintestinal disease symptoms; lesions of eyes, joints, skin, liver, and biliary tracts • Colon cancer (after 10 or more years of colitis) • Anemia resulting from intestinal blood loss and poor nutrient absorption	• Fluid and blood replacement as needed • Corticosteroids and sulfasalazine in colitis; possibly given with azathioprine to allow reduced corticosteroid dosages • Metronidazole in Crohn's disease • Surgical resection of affected area (total coloo tomy cures ulcerative colitis; Crohn's disease may recur in another segment following resection) • Nutritional support, possibly oral or parenteral hyperalimentation
Primary biliary cirrhosis	• Presence of mitochondrial antibody • Diminished suppressor cell function • Increased serum IgM levels • Inability to convert from IgM to IgG antibody synthesis • Complement-activating serum factor, possibly immune complexes • Granulomatous infiltrates in intrahepatic biliary tree • Markedly elevated serum alkaline phosphate levels	• Pruritus • Hyperlipidemia (especially hypercholesterolemia) with resulting xanthomas (yellowish lipid plaques in subcutaneous tissues) in periorbital areas, skin folds, and trauma sites • Steatorrhea and fat-soluble vitamin malabsorption after cholestasis develops, with resulting intestinal bile salt deficiency • Jaundice, dark urine, light stools • Anergy • Signs of portal hypertension and liver insufficiency • Metabolic bone disease with vertebral compression fractures	• Antihistamines, topical lotions, or cholestyramine for pruritus • Penicillamine for copper-chelating and anti-inflammatory effects • Cyclosporine A (investigational use only) • Substitution of dietary medium-chain triglycerides for long-chain triglycerides to reduce steatorrhea • Parenteral administration of fat-soluble vitamins D, A, and K • Plasmapheresis

Continued on page 44

Autoimmune Disorders

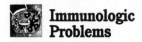

Organ-specific autoimmune disorders—*continued*

Disorder	Immunologic features and test findings	Signs and symptoms	Interventions
GASTROINTESTINAL—*continued*			
Primary biliary cirrhosis—*continued*	• Normal or slightly elevated serum transaminase levels • Elevated serum copper levels		
HEMATOLOGIC DISORDERS			
Idiopathic thrombocytopenic purpura	• Antiplatelet antibodies on platelets and in serum • Decreased platelet survival time • Depressed platelet count (acute, less than 30,000/mm³; chronic, 30,000 to 100,000/mm³) • Therapeutic response to prednisone and splenectomy	• Usually acute onset • Petechiae; ecchymoses; epistaxis; and gingival, gastrointestinal, or genitourinary bleeding • Possible cerebral hemorrhage • Acute systemic illness with fever (if thrombocytopenia is associated with another disease) • Splenomegaly likely • Moderate anemia resulting from blood loss and iron deficiency	• Precautions to reduce tissue trauma in patients prone to bleeding; for example, avoiding I.M. injections in patients with low platelet counts • Avoid administration of aspirin or other drugs that interfere with platelets or coagulation • Monitor vascular volume and oxygenation if severe bleeding occurs • Withdraw offending drug if drug-induced thrombocytopenia is suspected • In children, specific treatment often not needed. Corticosteroids given in severe thrombocytopenia and bleeding. • Splenectomy usually necessary in adults. Immunosuppressants given if splenectomy is ineffective.
Pernicious anemia	• Evidence of both humoral and cell-mediated immunity to gastric mucosal antigens • High incidence of antiparietal cell antibodies • Autoantibodies in gastric mucosal plasma cells and in secretions (IgA) • Parietal cell cytotoxicity	• Pallor, fatigue, progressive muscle weakness • Anorexia, weight loss • Neurologic involvement, including peripheral neuropathies, damage to pyramidal tract and posterior column neurons, and disturbances in higher cortical function • Macrocytic anemia and hypersegmentation of nuclei of neutrophil granulocytes, detected on peripheral blood smear • Megaloblastosis on examination of bone marrow aspirate • Serum B_{12} level below 120 pg/ml (normally 200 to 1500 pg/ml)	• Regular I.M. injections of vitamin B_{12} • Corticosteroid or immunosuppressant therapy (experimental)
Warm antibody autoimmune hemolytic anemia	• Positive direct antiglobulin (Coombs') test • Increased unconjugated serum bilirubin levels • Possibly associated with lymphoreticular malignancy or autoimmune disease	• Splenomegaly • Anemia and signs of hemolysis • Leukocytosis and thrombocytosis	• Treatment of underlying disease process • High-dose corticosteroid therapy • Splenectomy if corticosteroid therapy fails • Immunosuppressants if corticosteroids and splenectomy fail • Blood transfusion, if required, to prevent serious complication of anemia (avoid if possible because transfused blood is rapidly destroyed)

Autoimmune Disorders

Organ-specific autoimmune disorders—*continued*

Disorder	Immunologic features and test findings	Signs and symptoms	Interventions
NEUROLOGIC DISORDERS			
Multiple sclerosis	• Inflammatory demyelination of CNS white matter • Increased IgG level in cerebrospinal fluid (CSF), with oligoclonal bands • Elevated levels of antiviral antibodies in serum and CSF • Increased levels of IgG and myelin basic protein in CSF • Multiple sclerosis plaques visualized through magnetic resonance imaging • Abnormalities of immunoregulatory T cells	• Motor weakness, paresthesias • Impaired visual acuity, diplopia • Ataxia, urinary bladder dysfunction, impotence, spasticity • Acute exacerbations of signs and symptoms that persist for days to weeks with gradual recovery (more slowly in chronic, progressive disease) • Mild to moderate dementia (late)	• Symptomatic and supportive care • Corticosteroids, immunosuppressants, and plasmapheresis to shorten periods of exacerbation or arrest disease progress • Alpha-interferon and beta-interferon (investigational)
Myasthenia gravis	• Commonly associated with thymoma or thymic hyperplasia • Pathogenic autoantibodies directed against acetylcholine-receptor protein in serum • Other autoantibodies • Often associated with other autoimmune diseases	• Muscles often weak or normal at rest, becoming increasingly weaker with repetitive use. • Skeletal muscle weakness usually proximal, causing difficulty in climbing stairs, rising from chairs, combing hair, even holding head up • Weakness of extraocular muscles, manifested as diplopia or ptosis • Pharyngeal and facial muscle weakness resulting in dysphagia, dysarthria, and difficulty chewing	• Anticholinesterase drugs combined with atropine for long-term therapy • Thymectomy • Corticosteroids and immunosuppressants for patients unresponsive to anticholinesterase drugs or thymectomy • Plasmapheresis

Hypersensitivity Disorders: Four Types

Patricia Mosko, who contributed to this chapter, is a certified registered nurse practitioner at Temple University Hospital in Philadelphia. She received her BSN from La Salle University and her MSN from the University of Pennsylvania, both in Philadelphia.

Hypersensitivity refers to an exaggerated or inappropriate immune response that takes place after a second exposure to a particular antigen. Varying widely from person to person, hypersensitivity often causes inflammation and tissue damage. Severe hypersensitivity can even cause death.

In this chapter, we'll review the four types of hypersensitivity, how they can affect your patients, and how you should respond. But first, let's look at the body's normal response to an antigen.

Responding to an antigen

When the body encounters an antigen, it responds in phases. The first phase, initiated by exposure to the antigen, is called the *primary response.* At first, few or no antibodies appear in the serum. The immune system, though, recognizes the antigen as foreign and signals the appropriate cells to trigger antibody production. This *inductive* or *latent* phase is marked by cellular proliferation and differentiation. The duration of this phase depends upon the antigenicity (the ability of a substance to elicit an immune response), quantity, form, and solubility of the antigen, and the route of immunization. The sensitivity of the assay used to detect antibodies also plays a part in measuring the inductive phase. For example, antibodies can be detected 3 to 4 days after introduction of foreign erythrocytes (transfusion reaction), 5 to 7 days after introduction of soluble proteins, and 10 to 14 days after introduction of bacterial cells. During the early inductive phase, the IgM antibody (or immunoglobulin) predominates. However, IgM production is usually transient; within 2 weeks, IgG usually predominates.

A second exposure to the same antigen, even if it occurs years after the first, provokes a quicker, more aggressive response characterized by the rapid appearance of immunocompetent cells. Called the *secondary* (anamnestic or recall) *response*, this response owes its strength to the primary response, which created memory cells that become activated and respond rapidly when that same antigen reappears. What's more, circulating antibodies left over from the initial exposure can help drive the secondary response.

Typically, the secondary response develops faster than the primary one even if the amount of antigen diminishes sharply. However, if only a slight amount of antigen enters the body, the secondary response may not be activated. Instead, the antigen may be consumed in antigen-antibody complexes, phagocytized, and removed. If enough antigen remains after these local responses occur, the secondary response takes over. If exaggerated, this secondary response can cause hypersensitivity disorders.

The secondary response might also be produced by an antigen quite similar to the original. However, in this phenomenon, antibodies may not react quite as strongly as they would to the original antigen.

Types of hypersensitivity reactions

British immunologists R.R.A. Coombs and P.G. Gell classified hypersensitivity reactions into four types (I, II, III, and IV) based on immunologic pathogenesis. Antibodies mediate Types I, II, and III. Mainly T cells and macrophages mediate Type IV reactions.

Keep in mind that hypersensitivity can sometimes result from other reactions. For instance, IgA can activate the alternative pathway

Hypersensitivity Disorders

Hypersensitivity disorders: A quick review

Hypersensitivity type	Antibodies or cells involved	Effector cells	Mediators	Associated disorders
I Immediate	IgE	Mast cells Basophils	Histamine SRS-A ECF-A (others)	• Allergic rhinitis • Anaphylaxis • Extrinsic asthma
II Cytotoxic	IgG IgM	Polymorphonuclear leukocytes	Complement K cells	• Hemolytic disease of the newborn • Hyperacute graft rejection • Myasthenia gravis • Transfusion reactions
III Immune complex	IgG IgM	Polymorphonuclear leukocytes	Complement	• Arthus reaction • Rheumatoid arthritis • Serum sickness • Systemic lupus erythematosus
IV Cell-mediated	T cells	Mononuclear leukocytes	Lymphokines	• Contact dermatitis • Mycobacterial, protozoal, or fungal infections • Sarcoidosis • Tuberculosis

of the complement system, generating anaphylatoxins (C3a, C5a, C4a) that release mediators from mast cells. The result is a reaction similar to Type I hypersensitivity. Still other hypersensitivity reactions don't correlate with specific disorders. For the most part, the hypersensitivity reactions you see will be Types I and IV. (See *Hypersensitivity disorders: A quick review.*)

Type I hypersensitivity. Also known as immediate, anaphylactic, atopic, reaginic, or IgE-mediated hypersensitivity, this type of reaction generally develops immediately after contact with an antigen or allergen. Type I reactions are mediated almost exclusively by IgE antibodies. They include anaphylaxis, allergic rhinitis, extrinsic asthma, urticaria, angioedema, mastocytosis, and reactions to foods, drugs, and stinging insects. Atopy, a variety of Type I hypersensitivity, occurs only in certain predisposed or hypersensitive persons. (See *Atopy defined.*)

After the first exposure to an antigen, antibodies (usually IgE) form and bind to surface receptors on mast cells or basophils. These cells are now sensitized, setting the stage for a Type I reaction. When the same antigen reappears, it interacts with the bound IgE antibodies by cross-linking or bridging two IgE receptor molecules, thus activating a series of cellular reactions that trigger degranulation—the release of powerful chemical mediators. (See *Reviewing Type I hypersensitivity*, page 48.)

Mediators of Type I hypersensitivity include the following:
• histamine
• slow-reacting substance of anaphylaxis (SRS-A), also known as leukotrienes
• prostaglandins and thromboxanes
• eosinophil chemotactic factor of anaphylaxis (ECF-A)
• bradykinin
• serotonin
• platelet activating factor (PAF)

Continued on page 48

Atopy defined

Atopy refers to a genetic susceptibility to hypersensitivity rather than to a specific hypersensitivity response. Atopic patients usually display features of Type I hypersensitivity, such as asthma, eczema, hay fever, urticaria, a family history of allergy, and positive, immediate wheal-and-flare skin reactions to inhaled allergens.

An atopic reaction occurs in people genetically susceptible to such environmental allergens as pollen, mold, house dust, animal dander, and food. In hay fever, for instance, evidence suggests that genes closely linked to the human leukocyte antigen complex control the immune response. Upon exposure to the allergen, IgE antibodies form and trigger release of mediators—including histamine, slow-reacting substance of anaphylaxis, and eosinophil chemotactic factor of anaphylaxis—in the target organ, thereby prompting allergic symptoms.

Besides hay fever, atopic disorders include bronchial asthma, atopic dermatitis and, rarely, food allergy.

Hypersensitivity Disorders

Reviewing Type I hypersensitivity

On first exposure to an antigen, antibodies (usually IgE) form and bind to receptors, usually on the surface of mast cells or basophils. On second exposure, the antigen seeks out the bound IgE antibodies and links the two IgE receptor molecules on the sensitized cells. This causes mast cell degranulation and release of mediators.

IgE binds to mast cells via its Fc receptor. The cells are now sensitized.

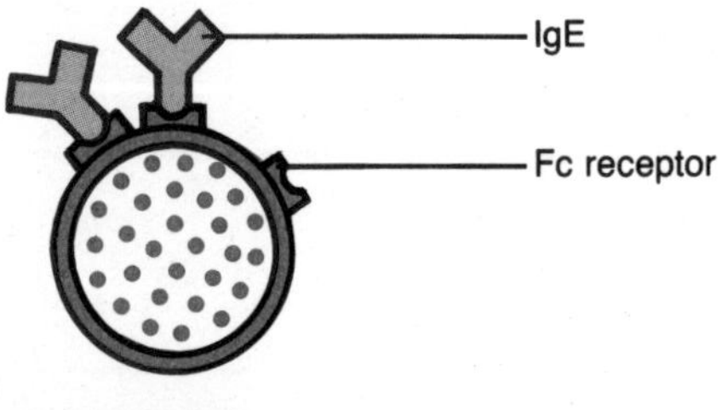

Antigen reaches the sensitized cells and binds to IgE, cross-linking the antibodies.

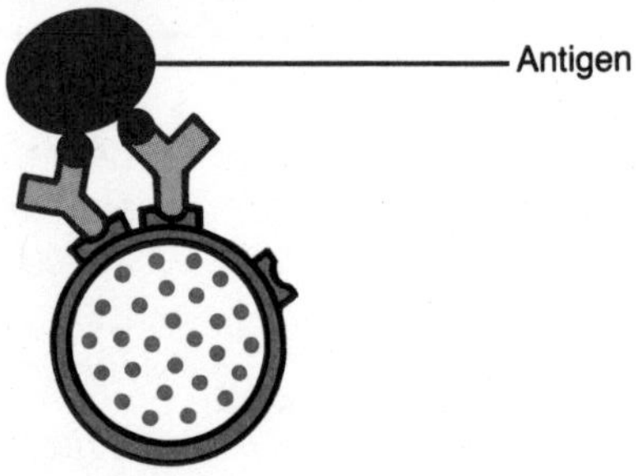

Mast cell degranulation occurs along with release of vasoactive amines and other mediators.

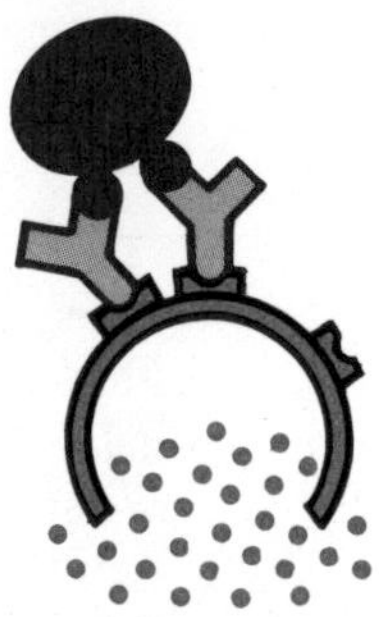

This leads to vasodilation, increased capillary permeability, smooth-muscle contraction, and eosinophilia.

Hypersensitivity reactions—*continued*

Histamine, the major chemical mediator of anaphylaxis, causes smooth muscle contraction, capillary dilation, increased capillary permeability, and reduced blood pressure. It also increases nasal and bronchial secretions and endothelial cell adhesiveness. Histamine's effects peak in 1 to 2 minutes and last about 10 minutes.

Hypersensitivity Disorders

For some time, researchers have recognized two histamine receptor types: H_1 and H_2. Stimulation of H_1 receptors dilates blood vessels, increases capillary permeability, and contracts nonvascular smooth muscles. Stimulation of H_2 receptors increases gastric acid secretions. The combined effects of H_1 and H_2 receptor stimulation probably cause vasodilation, possibly resulting in reduced blood pressure. Recently, researchers found a third histamine receptor (H_3) in the brain, lungs, skin, and spleen. Its function isn't known.

Capillary dilation, histamine's most characteristic effect, stems from direct action on vessels. Most apparent as facial and upper body flushing, dilation results from histamine's inhibitory effects on terminal arteriolar smooth muscle. Dilation in the venules, which lack smooth muscle, occurs mainly passively. Resistance declines in terminal arterioles and rises in histamine-constricted larger veins. By acting on the microcirculation, histamine triggers a chain of events that shifts plasma proteins and fluid from intravascular to extravascular compartments.

When released from basophils and mast cells, histamine causes an inflammatory response to tissue injury. Normally, inflammation develops only at the injury site. In anaphylaxis, however, this response affects the entire body.

The lipid *SRS-A*, another mediator of anaphylaxis, contracts bronchial smooth muscle and increases vascular permeability, thereby potentiating histamine's effects. It contains metabolites called leukotrienes (LTC_4, LTD_4, LTE_4), which play a part in asthmatic bronchospasm.

Prostaglandins may alter vascular permeability, contract smooth muscle, or enhance other mediator effects. *Thromboxanes* cause platelet aggregation. *ECF-A* prevents eosinophils from neutralizing other mediators and stimulates bradykinin and serotonin release.

Bradykinin, an extremely potent kinin (a polypeptide released during inflammation), stimulates smooth muscle contraction, including bronchoconstriction and vasoconstriction. It also increases capillary permeability and mucous membrane secretion.

Serotonin increases capillary permeability, especially in pulmonary capillaries, whereas *PAF* causes platelet release and aggregation.

Other mediators of anaphylaxis include high-molecular-weight neutrophil chemotactic factors and arachidonic acid metabolites.

Type II hypersensitivity. Also known as complement-dependent cytotoxicity, cytotoxic hypersensitivity, and antibody-dependent cytotoxic hypersensitivity, Type II hypersensitivity occurs when IgG, IgM, or both antibodies act against antigens found on host tissues or cell surfaces. These antibodies activate complement or cytotoxic action by killer (K) cells, thereby damaging target cells and possibly the surrounding tissue. (See *Reviewing Type II hypersensitivity*, page 50.)

Type II hypersensitivity disorders include transfusion reactions, hemolytic disease of the newborn, autoimmune hemolytic anemias, hyperacute graft rejection, Goodpasture's syndrome, and myasthenia gravis.

Continued on page 50

Hypersensitivity Disorders

Reviewing Type II hypersensitivity

In Type II hypersensitivity, antibodies act against cell-surface or tissue antigen. This reaction activates complement (C1q) and effector cells (killer cells), leading to cytotoxic effects against the body's own cells by complement-mediated lysis or killer (K) cells. Physiologic processes like phagocytosis, normally leveled against pathogenic microorganisms, become mechanisms of damage.

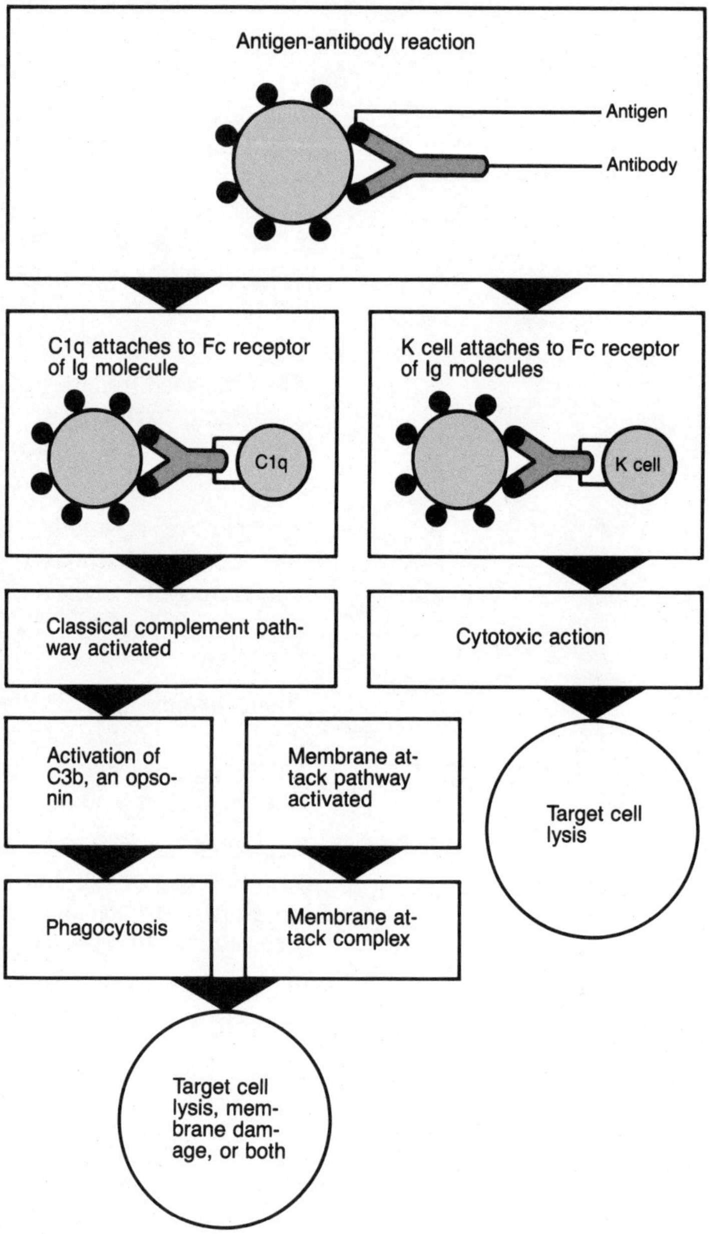

Hypersensitivity reactions—*continued*

Type III hypersensitivity. Also called immune complex, soluble complex, and toxic complex reactions, Type III hypersensitivity occurs when circulating immune complexes become deposited in host tissues. (IgG or IgM antibodies form circulating immune complexes with antigen and complement.) Normally, the mononuclear phagocyte system (MPS) removes these immune complexes; those that

Hypersensitivity Disorders

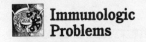

continue to circulate usually don't cause harm. However, if an immune complex becomes deposited in host tissue, it may activate complement-derived chemotactic factors, thus causing local tissue inflammation and damage. Type III hypersensitivity disorders include serum sickness, cryoglobulinemia, leprosy, malaria, hypersensitivity pneumonitis, acute glomerulonephritis and, locally, the Arthus reaction. (See *Reviewing Type III hypersensitivity*, page 52.)

Most of the time, increased vascular permeability probably triggers immune complex deposition. Immune complexes also tend to form in such high-blood-pressure sites as the glomerular capillaries, or in such turbulent sites as vessel bifurcations.

The precise location of deposition depends on the immune complex's size. In the kidney, for example, small immune complexes pass through the glomerular basement membrane, settling on the membrane's epithelial side. Large complexes can't cross the membrane and accumulate between the endothelium and the basement membrane or in the mesangium.

Disorders associated with immune complex formation fall into three groups. The first group stems from such persistent infections as staphylococcal infective endocarditis and viral hepatitis. Combined with a weak antibody response, these persistent low-grade infections can lead to chronic formation of immune complexes with eventual deposition, usually in the affected organ.

The second group stems from complications of autoimmune disease. Host tissues continually produce antibodies that act on "self" components (called autoantibodies). This leads to prolonged immune complex formation, overloading the MPS and encouraging immune complex deposition. Disorders in this group include systemic lupus erythematosus (SLE), rheumatoid arthritis, polyarteritis, Reiter's syndrome, giant cell arteritis, Wegener's granulomatosis, Henoch-Schönlein purpura, and polymyositis and dermatomyositis.

The third group stems from such inhaled allergens as molds, pollen, animal dander, and other plant and animal products. Repeated inhalation of these allergens can cause immune complex formation in the lungs or at other body surfaces.

Type IV hypersensitivity. Also called delayed, cellular, or cell-mediated hypersensitivity, Type IV hypersensitivity occurs when antigen trapped in macrophages can't be cleared. T cells sensitized from a previous encounter with that antigen then generate lymphokines, which mediate an inflammatory response by attracting macrophages to the site and amplifying the local response. (See *Reviewing Type IV hypersensitivity*, page 53.) Type IV hypersensitivity disorders stem from mycobacterial, protozoal, or fungal infections. They include blastomycosis, contact dermatitis, leishmaniasis, leprosy, listeriosis, sarcoidosis, schistosomiasis, and tuberculosis.

Type IV hypersensitivity reactions are divided into four categories: Jones-Mote, contact, tuberculin-type, and granulomatous. These reactions may exist alone, occur sequentially, or overlap.

Jones-Mote reaction. Regulated primarily by T-suppressor cells, this reaction occurs when soluble antigens induce basophils to infiltrate

Continued on page 54

Hypersensitivity Disorders

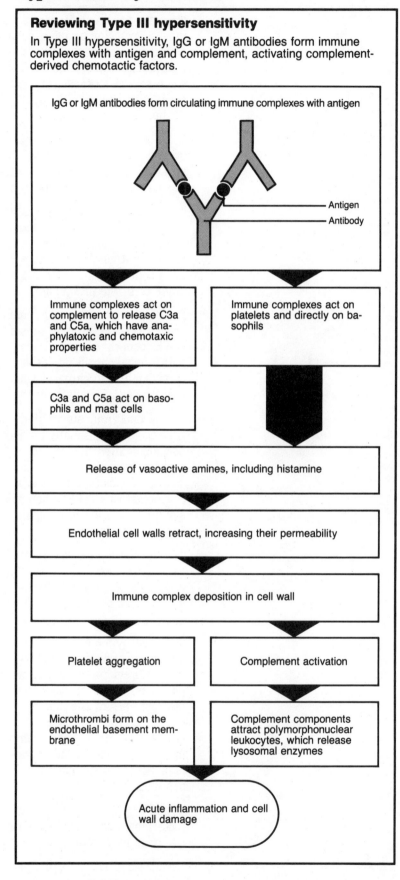

Reviewing Type III hypersensitivity

In Type III hypersensitivity, IgG or IgM antibodies form immune complexes with antigen and complement, activating complement-derived chemotactic factors.

IgG or IgM antibodies form circulating immune complexes with antigen

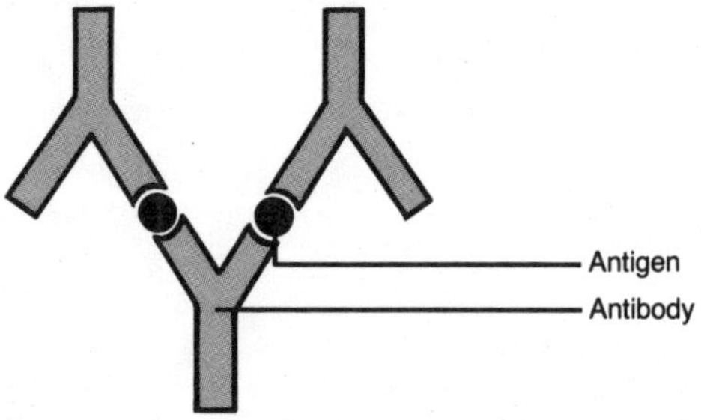

Immune complexes act on complement to release C3a and C5a, which have anaphylatoxic and chemotaxic properties

C3a and C5a act on basophils and mast cells

Immune complexes act on platelets and directly on basophils

Release of vasoactive amines, including histamine

Endothelial cell walls retract, increasing their permeability

Immune complex deposition in cell wall

Platelet aggregation

Microthrombi form on the endothelial basement membrane

Complement activation

Complement components attract polymorphonuclear leukocytes, which release lysosomal enzymes

Acute inflammation and cell wall damage

Hypersensitivity Disorders

Reviewing Type IV hypersensitivity

Type IV hypersensitivity occurs when macrophages fail to digest and clear antigens. Sensitized T cells, encountering an antigen for the second time, react by releasing lymphokines. Lymphokines activate an inflammatory reaction by attracting macrophages that release mediators, leading to cellular and tissue damage.

T cells are sensitized to antigen from previous exposure

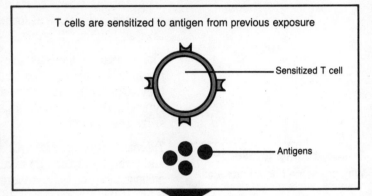

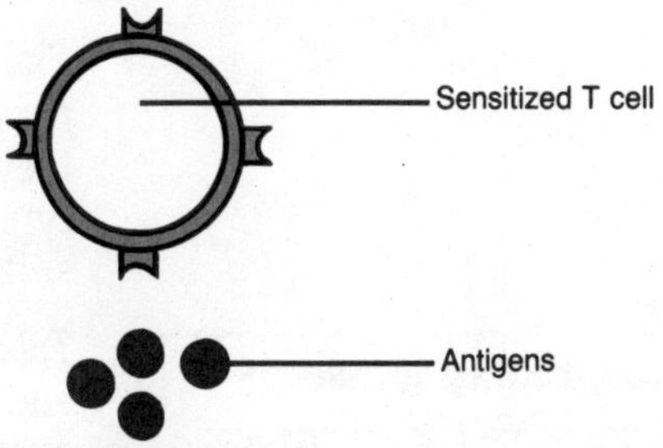

Antigen-presenting cell extends the antigen to sensitized T cell

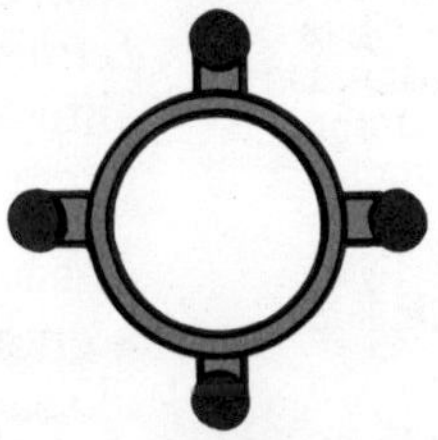

Sensitized T cell releases lymphokines, including macrophage activating factor

Macrophage activation

Inflammatory response

Release of intracellular products, such as lysozymes, leads to cellular and surrounding tissue damage

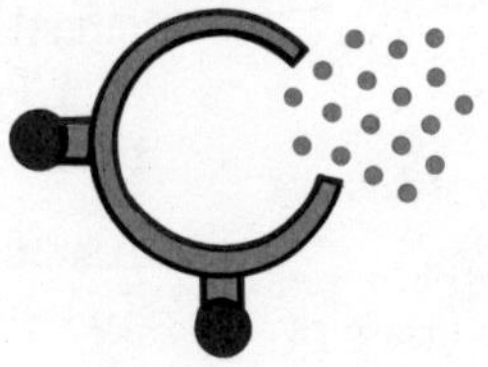

Hypersensitivity Disorders

Hypersensitivity reactions—*continued*

the area immediately under the epidermis. Although the peak response occurs 7 to 10 days after induction, skin swelling peaks in 24 hours. The reaction tends to disappear when antibodies appear.

Contact reaction. In this predominantly epidermal reaction, eczema erupts at the site of contact with an antigen, commonly poison ivy or poison oak. The response usually peaks in 48 hours, but may take as long as 72 hours.

The causative haptens are substances of low molecular weight normally unable to produce an immune response on their own. But they apparently cross the skin and bind with carrier molecules, typically the host's serum proteins. These molecules can then sensitize the patient.

Tuberculin-type reactions. Characterized by local dermal induration and swelling at the site of antigen contact caused by infiltration of mononuclear cells, a tuberculin-type reaction may also produce fever. It usually peaks in 48 hours, but may take up to 72 hours.

This reaction may occur in hypersensitive people after exposure to such soluble antigens as *Mycobacterium tuberculosis*, *M. leprae*, and *Leishmania tropica*. It may also occur from exposure to nonmicrobial antigens. In some cases, a tuberculin-type reaction could develop into a granulomatous reaction after 21 to 28 days.

Granulomatous reaction. The most severe Type IV hypersensitivity, a granulomatous reaction is characterized by indurated skin granulomas that usually peak about 4 weeks after exposure; however, they may peak in as little as 14 days in some patients. Granulomatous hypersensitivity is responsible for many pathologic effects in disorders involving T cell–mediated immunity. It may result from:
- the inability of macrophages to kill ingested microbes or other organic substances, leading to the continued presence of foreign substances within macrophages
- the inability of macrophages to digest inorganic substances, such as talc
- the continued presence of immune complexes, such as in allergic alveolitis
- sensitization to such microbial antigens as *Mycobacterium tuberculosis* and *M. leprae*
- zirconium sensitivity
- sarcoidosis.

Hypersensitivity types I, II, III, and IV don't always occur in isolation. What's more, a disorder may fit under more than one classification. For example, researchers may classify myasthenia gravis as a Type II disorder, an autoimmune disorder, or a musculoskeletal disorder.

Assessment

To determine if hypersensitivity has caused your patient's disorder, start by thoroughly investigating his chief complaint, any related signs and symptoms, and his personal and family history. (See *Susceptibility to allergy*.)

First, you'll need a complete account of the patient's symptoms, which may range from a rash to hypovolemic shock and respiratory

Susceptibility to allergy

Why are some people prone to allergies, while others never suffer a sniffle or a sneeze? Genetic factors are one reason. Scientists have isolated genes controlling antigenic specificity, immune response intensity, and the class of responding immunoglobulins. Unknown factors controlling target organ localization and clinical expression are another reason. Scientists, though, haven't yet identified the genes controlling target organ localization.

The allergen's quantity and exposure route may also affect sensitization and possible symptoms. For instance, a patient suffering from a viral respiratory infection may experience a heightened response to an inhaled allergen.

Keep in mind that an allergy-associated disorder (such as asthma, atopic dermatitis, anaphylaxis, angioedema, contact dermatitis, drug-induced cytolysis, rhinitis, and urticaria) may arise through nonimmunologic mechanisms. In some instances, a disorder develops without an external trigger, such as in nonallergic asthma.

Drugs and other agents may also arouse mediators of inflammation nonimmunologically. In fact, researchers have been unable to identify specific allergens to explain these reactions:
- nonspecific histamine release by opiates, a direct mast cell effect
- asthma caused by aspirin, possibly an aberrant metabolism of arachidonic acid
- asthma caused by inhaled isocyanates
- anaphylactoid reactions from iodinated contrast media
- urticaria from shellfish and berries.

Hypersensitivity Disorders

distress. Keep in mind that, in an emergency, you may need to intervene as you obtain the history.

As you collect information, be alert for clues to hypersensitivity. Ask your patient the following questions. (Even though the term "allergy" refers only to hypersensitivity Types I and IV, use it to refer broadly to hypersensitivity.)

- What symptoms do you have now and how did you notice them?
- Do you have allergies?
- Does anyone in your family have allergies?
- Do your symptoms vary over the course of the day? The week? The month? The year?
- Do they seem worse in a particular location? At home? In school or the office? In the car?
- What pets do you have?
- What hobbies do you have?
- How does the weather affect your symptoms?
- What medications do you take regularly? Do you use any recreational drugs?
- Does your skin react to any plants, perfumes, cosmetics, or topical drugs?
- Did you change your diet just before you noticed the symptoms?

Diagnostic tests. Diagnosing a hypersensitivity disorder (and gauging potential response to treatment) may require one or more tests. General tests of hypersensitivity include serum, skin, and provocation tests.

Serum tests. These include the white blood cell (WBC) count and differential, serum IgE level, radioallergosorbent test (RAST), and enzyme-linked immunosorbent assay (ELISA).

The WBC count and differential includes an eosinophil count. Eosinophils normally make up 1% to 3% of circulating WBCs; in allergic patients, eosinophils may make up 10% to 20%. A count above 350 to 400 cells/mm^3 is considered abnormal.

Serum IgE rises in hypersensitivity, especially in Type I. Normal adult levels are about 250 ng/ml (or about 90 IU/ml, with a range of 29 to 800 IU/ml).

RAST and ELISA detect IgE or IgG antibodies in serum; however, they're somewhat less sensitive than skin tests.

Skin tests. Initially, a prick test or a scratch test is usually performed to detect IgE antibodies. To perform the prick test, use a needle to apply a drop of concentrated allergen extract to the back or the volar surface of the patient's arm; then prick the skin directly under the drop. To perform the scratch test, make a short, linear scratch in the skin, and then apply the allergen. For both methods, wipe off the allergen after 20 minutes and quantify and record the reaction. Consider a reaction of 2+ or more to be significant. (See *Gauging reactions to skin tests.*)

If these tests yield questionable results, you may need to perform a more sensitive intracutaneous test that also detects IgE antibodies. As ordered, administer the control dose. Then inject no more than 0.01 ml (preferably 0.005 ml) of sterile allergen extract intradermally into the lateral upper arm or the volar portion of the

Continued on page 56

Gauging reactions to skin tests

For the prick test and scratch test, use this rating scale:
- Negative: Absence of wheal or erythema
- 1+: Absence of wheal; erythema of less than 20 mm in diameter
- 2+: Absence of wheal; erythema exceeds 20 mm in diameter
- 3+: Wheal with erythema
- 4+: Wheal with pseudopods and erythema.

For the intracutaneous test, use this scale:
- Negative: Same characteristics as control
- 1+: Wheal double the size of the control; erythema of less than 20 mm in diameter
- 2+: Wheal double the size of the control; erythema exceeds 20 mm in diameter
- 3+: Wheal triple the size of the control; erythema present
- 4+: Wheal with pseudopods and erythema.

Hypersensitivity Disorders

Hypersensitivity reactions—*continued*

forearm. In 20 minutes, read the reaction. A response of 2+ or greater constitutes a positive reaction. Keep in mind that injection of excessive amounts of some allergens will give a false-positive reaction. Carefully determine the correct concentration for each allergen.

To detect IgG antibodies, use the Arthus reaction as a gauge. As ordered, inject 0.1 ml of sterilized allergen extract intradermally and read the reaction 5 to 8 hours later. Induration, usually with tenderness and erythema, indicates a positive reaction.

Two other skin tests, used to detect T cell–mediated hypersensitivity, include the tuberculin skin test and the patch test. To perform the tuberculin test (also known as the delayed hypersensitivity skin reaction), inject 0.1 ml of test solution intradermally and note the reaction after 24, 48, and 72 hours. Erythema and induration measuring 5 mm or more after 24 to 48 hours constitute a positive test.

Expect to perform the patch test to detect T cell–mediated hypersensitivity in allergic contact dermatitis. To perform an open patch test, simply apply the appropriate dilution of the test allergen to the skin. To perform a closed patch test, apply the allergen, cover the area with a patch, and secure with tape. In both tests, note the reaction after 48 hours. Erythema, papules, or vesicles constitute a positive test. To obtain a photoallergic contact reaction (photo patch test), expose the skin to ultraviolet light or sunlight after removing the patch.

Provocation tests. As the name suggests, provocation tests are used to elicit and thus identify an allergic reaction under controlled conditions. Typically, a positive provocation test doesn't prove that allergy caused a hypersensitivity reaction but, along with the patient's history and other test results, it can aid diagnosis.

To detect respiratory allergens, assess the patient's response after he inhales increasing concentrations of allergen suspended in solution and aerosolized through a nebulizer. To detect food allergies, tell the patient to keep a food diary for at least a week. Then he should stop eating the foods he most suspects as allergens and wait for his symptoms to subside. Then, one at a time, he should reintroduce foods to his diet, observing for an immediate or delayed reaction that will identify the allergen.

Anaphylaxis

A systemic form of immediate hypersensitivity, anaphylaxis causes immediate and dramatic vascular and bronchial changes leading to profound hypovolemia and severe respiratory distress. Without prompt diagnosis and intervention, it may cause death.

Most commonly, anaphylaxis is mediated by IgE and accompanied by release of histamine and leukotrienes. However, in most anaphylactoid reactions, IgG-mediated or IgM-mediated complement-dependent mechanisms generate anaphylatoxins or kinins. (See *Understanding anaphylactoid reactions.*)

Understanding anaphylactoid reactions

Although anaphylactoid reactions cause signs of anaphylaxis, they don't involve an allergen–IgE antibody interaction. These reactions arise through nonimmunologic release of vasoactive and inflammatory mediators in susceptible individuals. They may be triggered by such nonprotein substances as I.V. radiographic contrast media, aspirin, and chymopapain.

Anaphylactoid reactions require the same treatment as anaphylaxis.

Hypersensitivity Disorders

Common allergens

Antigens that give rise to Type I hypersensitivity, allergens include any foreign substance capable of eliciting an immune response. These primarily include complex organic chemicals, especially proteins. In contrast, simple organic chemicals and inorganic compounds and metals more commonly cause cell-mediated allergies.

Some foreign substances are more likely to be allergenic than others. The following allergens commonly cause anaphylaxis:
- protein drugs (presumably complete antigens)—incompatible blood, vaccines, allergen extracts, enzymes
- nonprotein drugs (presumably haptens)—penicillins and other antibiotics, sulfonamides, local anesthetics, salicylates
- foods—legumes (especially peanuts), nuts, berries, seafood, egg albumin
- stinging insects—honeybees, wasps, hornets, yellow jackets, red ants.

Besides its systemic form, anaphylaxis may strike specific tissues, including the GI tract, nasal mucosa, or skin. Almost any allergen can cause an anaphylactic or anaphylactoid reaction. (See *Common allergens.*)

Allergens may enter the body through:
- injection (drugs, serum, contrast media, and insect or animal venom)
- ingestion (foods and drugs)
- inhalation (drugs, chemicals, pollens)
- skin contact (drugs, chemicals).

An all-or-nothing response, anaphylaxis depends on many factors, including:
- *Amount of allergen.* A small amount may not cause anaphylaxis. For example, a wasp sting may deliver too little venom to cause anaphylaxis.
- *Absorption rate.* Delayed absorption of an ingested allergen may keep its concentration too low to cause a reaction.
- *Predisposition.* For example, a person with asthma or atopy (hypersensitivity) has an increased anaphylaxis risk and may develop it from even a minute allergen dose.
- *Antibody levels.* After a number of years, antibody levels gradually decline. Eventually, even a high-risk individual may have too few antibodies to produce anaphylaxis.
- *Allergen's chemical makeup.* Soluble antigens produce the most overwhelming reaction, usually within a few minutes. Soluble antigens include such I.V. agents as contrast media, analgesics, and antibiotics.
- *Entry site.* For example, an insect sting in a highly vascular area, such as the lips, can produce a response within minutes.

Anaphylaxis follows the pathogenesis of a Type I hypersensitivity reaction. Initial exposure to an antigen occurs during the sensitization phase. The immune system forms antibodies, usually IgE, that bind to receptors on mast cells or basophils. At this point, the mast cells or basophils remain inactive. After 3 to 5 days, antibody levels are usually sufficient to produce anaphylaxis if a second exposure to the same antigen occurs.

The next antigen exposure brings on the second phase of anaphylaxis: mediator release. The antigen interacts with IgE antibodies on basophils and on tissue-fixed mast cells, especially in the lungs, bronchial smooth muscle, and vascular endothelium, causing degranulation of mast cells and basophils. The subsequent release of chemical mediators produces the signs and symptoms of anaphylaxis. (See *Mast cell degranulation*, page 58).

Release of some chemical mediators may trigger release of other mediators, such as those of the complement system. This causes further physiologic damage, which exacerbates anaphylaxis.

Complications of anaphylaxis include laryngeal edema, respiratory failure, shock, or cardiac dysrhythmias that may be fatal. On rare occasions, irreversible shock can persist for hours. Permanent brain damage may result from hypoxia caused by respiratory or cardiovascular failure. Urticaria or angioedema may recur for months after anaphylaxis caused by penicillin.

Continued on page 58

Hypersensitivity Disorders

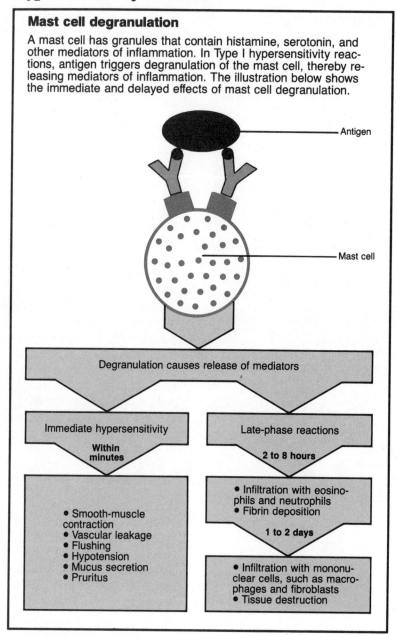

Mast cell degranulation

A mast cell has granules that contain histamine, serotonin, and other mediators of inflammation. In Type I hypersensitivity reactions, antigen triggers degranulation of the mast cell, thereby releasing mediators of inflammation. The illustration below shows the immediate and delayed effects of mast cell degranulation.

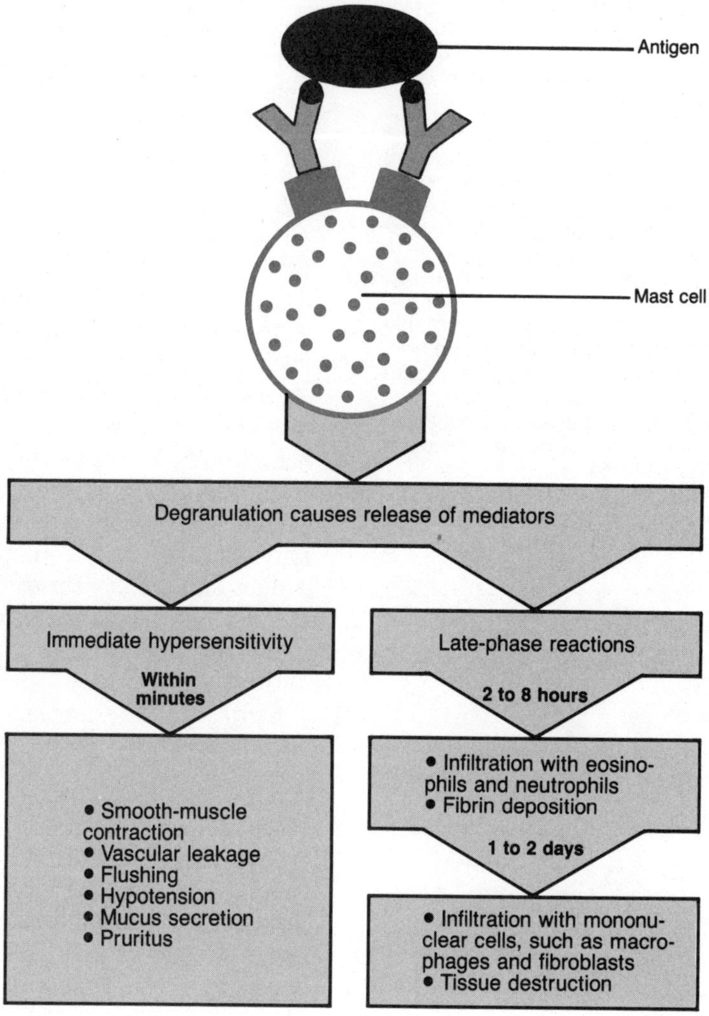

Anaphylaxis—*continued*

Assessment

Consider anaphylaxis a possible cause for any unexplained acute respiratory distress. The patient's history can provide crucial information about recent exposure to a potential antigen. Note the time from exposure to symptom onset—although serious, reactions occurring more than 2 hours after exposure don't qualify as anaphylaxis. Remember that anaphylaxis means *immediate* hypersensitivity.

If you suspect anaphylaxis, be prepared to intervene as you assess the patient. Death from anaphylaxis most frequently stems from asphyxiation secondary to bronchoconstriction. To prevent asphyxiation, continually assess your patient's respiratory status. If his condition permits, ask him about any allergies or atopy, such as asthma. Try to find out whether he's had similar reactions before

Hypersensitivity Disorders

and, if so, to which substance. A patient who's had an anaphylactic reaction to one substance may react the same way to a chemically similar antigen. If the patient can't respond to your questions, ask any bystanders or family members about his history and look for a medical identification tag or wallet card.

Determine if the patient took any medications during the hour preceding the appearance of symptoms. Specifically ask about any emergency medication (perhaps from an anaphylaxis kit) or administration of a beta blocker, such as propranolol. Beta blockers may inhibit the action of epinephrine, the main anaphylaxis treatment.

Signs and symptoms depend upon the allergen's entry route, the amount of allergen absorbed, the rate of absorption, and the degree of patient hypersensitivity. For example, a sensitized person may develop localized pruritic urticaria at an insect sting or drug injection site before experiencing severe systemic symptoms.

The most lethal reactions typically occur within minutes of exposure to the offending agent. The victim may experience chest tightness or a feeling of impending doom, possibly without preceding symptoms. Generalized skin signs—diffuse erythema, flushing, urticaria, and periorbital and mouth angioedema—may precede severe, rapidly progressive respiratory distress (caused by laryngeal edema and bronchospasm). The posterior pharynx, vocal cords, and uvula commonly become swollen and edematous. Auscultation may reveal diffuse wheezes and prolonged expirations. Hypotension and other signs of shock may follow, although such signs sometimes occur first. Changes in level of consciousness usually parallel respiratory effects: initial alertness gives way to decreased responsiveness as the patient's arterial oxygen (PaO_2) level or cerebral perfusion declines. (See *How anaphylaxis develops,* page 60.)

Diagnostic tests. The doctor will rely on history and physical findings rather than on specific tests to diagnose anaphylaxis. However, serum and skin tests may be performed after recovery to help determine appropriate preventative therapy and future treatment.

Planning

Before planning your nursing care, develop the nursing diagnosis by identifying the patient's actual or potential problem, then relating it to its cause. Possible nursing diagnoses for a patient with anaphylaxis include:

- gas exchange, impaired; related to bronchoconstriction
- anxiety; related to inadequate gas exchange
- tissue perfusion, alteration in (cerebral); related to hypovolemia
- cardiac output, alteration in (decreased); related to hypovolemia
- fluid volume, alteration in (deficit); related to increased capillary permeability
- knowledge deficit (allergy); related to inadequate patient teaching
- coping, ineffective individual; related to unexpected hospitalization.

The sample nursing care plan on page 61 shows expected outcomes, nursing interventions, and discharge planning for one nursing diagnosis listed above. However, you'll want to tailor each care plan to fit your patient's needs.

Continued on page 60

Hypersensitivity Disorders

How anaphylaxis develops

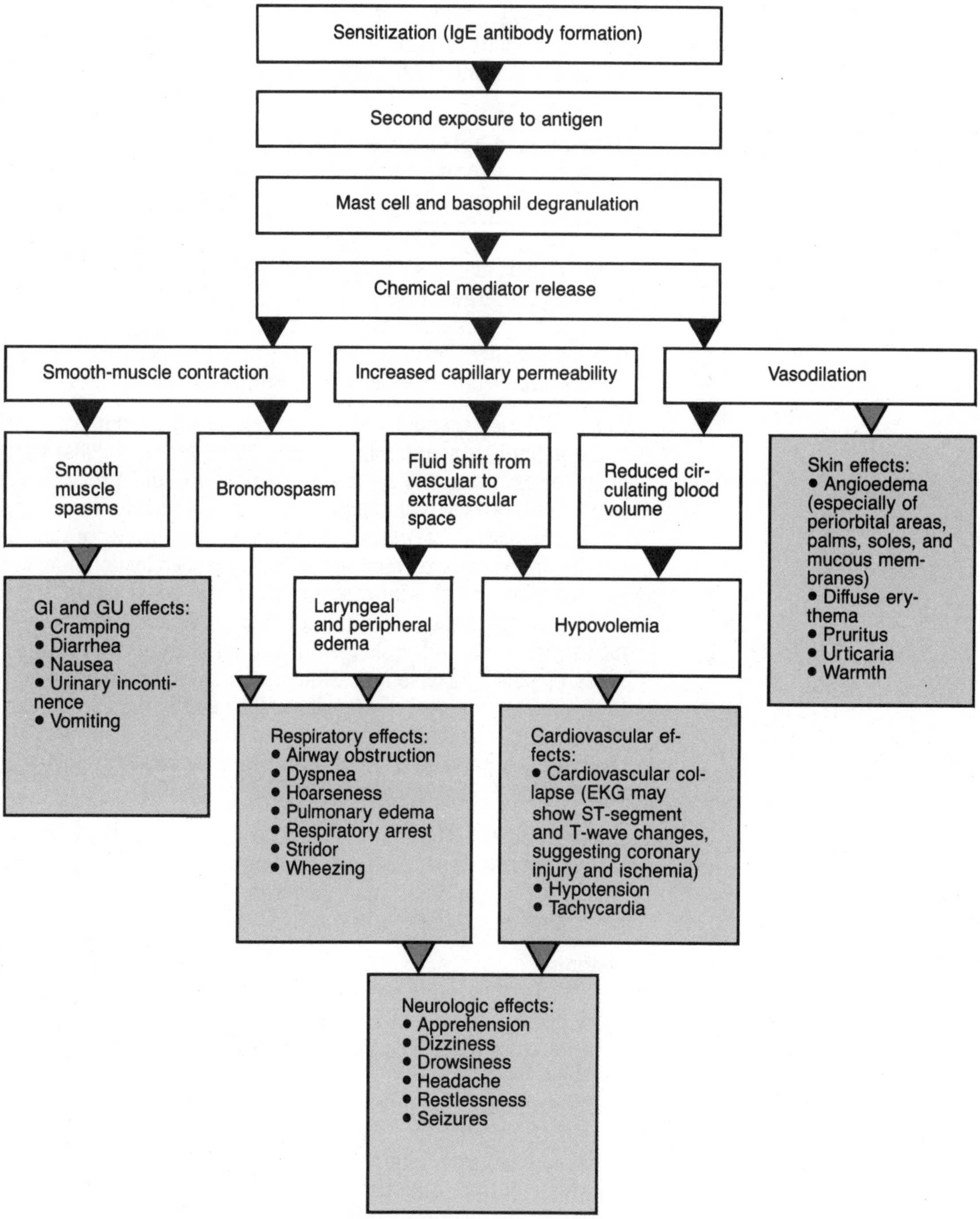

Anaphylaxis—*continued*

Intervention

Regardless of how severe anaphylaxis becomes, treatment goals always include:

- providing ventilation
- restoring adequate circulation
- preventing recurrence.

Remember, your patient's condition may change rapidly, so be sure to assess him continuously as you intervene.

Hypersensitivity Disorders

Sample nursing care plan: Anaphylaxis

Nursing diagnosis	Expected outcomes
Gas exchange, impaired; related to bronchoconstriction	The patient will: • maintain adequate gas exchange. • show reduced respiratory effort. • show no signs of wheezing.
Nursing interventions	**Discharge planning**
• Ensure airway patency; have emergency airway equipment nearby. • Help the patient find a position that promotes effective breathing and reduces oxygen consumption. • Evaluate effectiveness of oxygen therapy, if needed; notify doctor of any changes. • Assess and record vital signs and auscultate breath sounds, as indicated. • Monitor hemoglobin, hematocrit, and arterial blood gas levels; notify doctor of any abnormalities.	• Discuss disorder with patient and family. Reinforce treatment and care plan. • Encourage patient to wear a medical identification tag notifying others of his allergy. • Teach patient and family how to recognize signs of anaphylaxis. • Arrange for follow-up care, if indicated. • Teach patient and family how to use anaphylaxis kit, if needed. • Inform the patient when to seek medical attention. • Tell the patient and caregivers how to contact emergency medical services.

Providing ventilation. Maintain airway patency and be prepared to intervene with airway control measures or to assist with artificial airway placement (endotracheal intubation or tracheotomy, for example). As ordered, give high oxygen concentrations to help protect vital organ function. Watch for signs of laryngeal edema.

Take immediate measures to promote ventilation and reduce oxygen demand. For example, help the patient into a comfortable position and tell him to inhale slowly and exhale through pursed lips, if possible.

While ensuring ventilatory adequacy, try to prevent further exposure to the causative agent; such exposure will exacerbate the patient's condition. For anaphylaxis caused by I.V. drugs or contrast media, stop the drugs or procedure immediately. For venom-induced anaphylaxis, apply a tourniquet to the patient's arm or leg above the sting, if appropriate. Some doctors advocate removing the stinger by scraping the site with a dull object, because grasping and pulling could contract the venom sac and release more toxin.

Besides supporting ventilation, expect to administer drugs to block or counteract histamine's effects. *Epinephrine*, the preferred drug:
- constricts dilated vessels (alpha stimulation) to counteract hypotension and vasodilation
- increases heart rate and improves myocardial contractility to counteract cardiovascular collapse
- dilates bronchioles (beta stimulation) to counteract bronchoconstriction
- inhibits histamine release and negates the effects of circulating histamine to reverse histamine-related bronchiolar constriction, vasodilation, and edema
- prevents further mast cell or basophil degranulation.

Epinephrine's dosage and administration route depend on the patient's condition. In early anaphylaxis, the doctor may order S.C. or I.M. injection of 0.3 to 0.5 ml of a 1:1,000 solution (0.01 ml/kg for a child). However, if the patient's in acute respiratory distress, expect to give up to 5 ml of a 1:10,000 epinephrine solution I.V. If

Continued on page 62

Hypersensitivity Disorders

Immunotherapy

Also called allergy desensitization or hyposensitization, immunotherapy is most commonly used for allergic rhinitis, allergic asthma, and Hymenoptera insect sting anaphylaxis. In this therapy, the patient receives gradually increasing doses of an extract containing allergens that would normally produce symptoms. Prolonged therapy attempts to alter the patient's immune response and thereby reduce allergic symptoms.

During the initial months of treatment, serum IgE levels rise slightly. Over the next several years, they gradually fall to below pretreatment levels. Rarely, however, does treatment produce complete desensitization by eliminating circulating IgE. Instead, it induces formation of a blocking antibody—an IgG antibody specific for the injected allergen. This antibody binds with circulating allergen without initiating a Type I reaction.

Most patients receive either perennial immunotherapy or preseasonal immunotherapy. In the perennial method, the patient initially receives injections once or twice a week at doses low enough to avoid a local or systemic reaction. The dose gradually increases until reaching the highest level the patient can tolerate without excessive local or systemic reactions (the maintenance dose). He'll continue to receive this maintenance dose at less frequent intervals, usually every 2 to 6 weeks, depending upon his response.

In the preseasonal method, immunotherapy begins 3 to 6 months before pollen season. The patient receives gradually increasing doses until just before the season begins.

Expect to inject the allergens subcutaneously on the lateral or dorsal portion of the upper arm. After injection, observe for a systemic reaction for 20 minutes. If one occurs, notify the doctor immediately. With maintenance doses, most patients experience local swelling 3 to 4 mm in diameter, erythema, and pruritus that lasts less than 24 hours.

Anaphylaxis—*continued*

vascular collapse prevents venous access, give epinephrine endotracheally, or inject it into the vascular tissue beneath the tongue, as ordered.

Because epinephrine's action lasts only 3 to 5 minutes, the patient may need repeated doses if he doesn't respond rapidly. To help assess the drug's effect on heart rhythm, begin continuous cardiac monitoring, as ordered.

If the patient's receiving a beta blocker, such as propranolol, he may not respond to customary epinephrine doses. If he gets no relief within 2 minutes after receiving epinephrine, expect the doctor to increase the dose, the frequency of administration, or both.

If bronchoconstriction persists despite initial relief from epinephrine, the doctor may order I.V. *aminophylline*, a bronchodilator with a longer duration of action. Like epinephrine, aminophylline helps block additional mast cell and basophil degranulation.

Antihistamines like diphenhydramine usually don't relieve severe bronchoconstriction, but they can help counteract peripheral effects, such as pruritus. Cimetidine may be used to treat urticaria.

Corticosteroids may be used as supportive therapy. These drugs stabilize capillary walls, reduce fluid shifts by reducing capillary permeability, maintain blood pressure, and minimize further systemic reactions by halting degranulation.

Restoring adequate circulation. Once you've ensured the patient's ventilation, expect to begin fluid replacement to correct intravascular fluid loss from third-space shifts and vasodilation. As ordered, insert I.V. lines and administer crystalloid solutions, colloid solutions, or both. Titrate fluid doses according to your patient's blood pressure and perfusion status. *Important:* Watch carefully for signs of fluid overload, which may cause serious complications.

The doctor may order a vasopressor, such as norepinephrine or dopamine, if fluid therapy fails to maintain adequate blood pressure. Vasopressors improve cardiac contractility and counteract vasodilation. However, because these drugs cause vasoconstriction, they may further compromise tissue perfusion. Monitor your patient carefully if he's receiving a vasopressor.

Placing the patient in a Trendelenburg's or supine position may also help circulation. However, be careful not to compromise ventilation.

A terrifying experience, anaphylaxis can increase your patient's heart rate and oxygen demands. Calm him by providing continuous emotional support. Explain that he's having an allergic reaction, and assure him that you and other health care workers will monitor him closely and treat him appropriately. Explain procedures as you perform them, answer his questions, and don't hesitate to touch him reassuringly.

Preventing recurrence. When the patient stabilizes, continue observing him for several hours, watching for indications of delayed reaction to anaphylaxis or its treatment. Instruct him to avoid any vasodilatory stimulation (such as from vasodilatory drugs, alcohol, and hot showers or baths) for at least 24 hours.

Hypersensitivity Disorders

Anaphylaxis kits

Here are some of the kits available to patients at risk for anaphylaxis:
- *Ana-Kit* (Hollister-Stier Laboratories) includes two 0.3-mg doses of epinephrine 1:1,000 in a 1-ml disposable sterile syringe; four chewable 2-mg tablets of chlorpheniramine maleate; two sterile alcohol pads; and a tourniquet.
- *EpiPen Auto-Injector* (Center Labs) delivers a 0.3-mg I.M. dose of epinephrine 1:1,000 in a 2-ml disposable injector.
- *EpiPen Jr. Auto-Injector* (Center Labs) delivers a 0.15-mg I.M. dose of epinephrine 1:2,000 in a 2-ml disposable injector.

Once the causative agent's been identified, instruct the patient to avoid substances likely to cause future reactions. The doctor may recommend immunotherapy (also called desensitization) to alleviate allergic reactions and reduce the risk of future episodes. (See *Immunotherapy*.) In this therapy, introduction of small amounts of antigen gradually exhausts antibodies bound to mast cells or basophils. The body then can't release enough chemical mediators to cause anaphylaxis.

Advise the patient to wear an identification tag or bracelet that lists allergens to which he's sensitive. Also urge him to carry a wallet card describing his allergic sensitivities. If he can't avoid potential anaphylactic agents, such as bee venom, he may need a prophylactic antihistamine, a sympathomimetic drug, or both to reduce the severity of any future reactions. Suggest that he obtain an anaphylaxis kit so he can give himself epinephrine injections. (See *Anaphylaxis kits*.)

To help prevent anaphylaxis in any patient, ask about known allergies or a history of anaphylactic reactions. Be sure to document the information in the patient's record.

Evaluation
Base your evaluation on the expected outcomes listed on your nursing care plan. To help determine whether your patient's improved, ask yourself the following questions:
- Has the patient's breathing improved?
- Is he able to maintain adequate gas exchange?
- Are his arterial blood gas levels within the normal range?
- Are his breath sounds normal? Does auscultation reveal wheezes?

The answers to these questions will help you evaluate the effectiveness of your patient's care and determine his future needs. Keep in mind that these questions stem from the care plan on page 61. Your questions may differ.

Other selected hypersensitivity disorders

The complexity of the immune response makes it impossible to discuss all hypersensitivity disorders in a single chapter. On the following pages, you'll find discussions of selected disorders. They include:
- Type I hypersensitivity disorders—allergic rhinitis, allergic asthma, urticaria and angioedema, hereditary angioedema, and atopic dermatitis.
- Type II hypersensitivity disorders—hemolytic disease of the newborn.
- Type IV hypersensitivity disorders—sarcoidosis.

For examples of Type III disorders, turn to the discussion of autoimmune disorders in Chapter 2.

Allergic rhinitis
The most common atopic reaction to inhaled allergens, allergic rhinitis (or hay fever) strikes people of any age but usually first occurs during childhood or adolescence. Symptoms may recur throughout life; their severity depends upon the extent of allergen exposure.

Continued on page 64

Hypersensitivity Disorders

Selected hypersensitivity disorders—*continued*

Assessment. Look for the following signs and symptoms when assessing allergic rhinitis:
- profuse, watery rhinorrhea
- paroxysmal sneezing
- nasal obstruction
- itching of the nose and palate
- intense itching of the conjunctiva and eyelids
- conjunctivitis, unaccompanied by nasal symptoms
- an absence of fever
- headache.

The patient may also complain of:
- malaise
- muscle soreness, following an intense period of sneezing.

Ask the patient when his symptoms occur. Symptoms of pollen allergy, for instance, occur seasonally. Symptoms of sensitivity to a perennial allergen, such as house dust, may occur year round. Multiple allergies may bring about perennial symptoms with seasonal exacerbations.

Diagnostic tests. Diagnosis hinges on the patient history and physical findings during the symptomatic phase, including nasal and serum eosinophilia. Serum IgE may be normal or slightly elevated. To detect specific sensitivities, expect to administer skin tests.

Intervention. Advise the patient to avoid allergen exposure. The doctor may treat allergic rhinitis with immunotherapy or drug therapy. Most likely, drug therapy for allergic rhinitis will include antihistamines. Nasal decongestants may be prescribed alone or along with antihistamines. Sympathomimetic eye drops may alleviate allergic conjunctivitis. Cromolyn nasal spray or eyedrops may benefit some patients. Corticosteroids may effectively relieve symptoms; however, give them with extreme care because they heighten susceptibility to infection.

Urticaria and angioedema

Both common reactions, allergic urticaria and angioedema are localized, cutaneous forms of anaphylaxis. Possibly appearing simultaneously, these reactions may be provoked by the same or similar allergens that cause anaphylaxis and induced by similar immunologic mechanisms.

Usually acute, self-limiting, and episodic, urticaria may take a chronic or recurrent form. Localized increases in vascular permeability result in multiple, well-demarcated areas of skin swelling, usually accompanied by pruritus and restricted to areas of skin trauma or pressure. Angioedema is similar, but affects deeper blood vessels, causing diffuse swelling, usually without pruritus.

Assessment. Take a thorough food and drug history. Ingested allergens cause urticaria more frequently than inhalants. Ask about environmental factors and recent emotional stress. Be aware of these possible causes:
- Physical factors. Most commonly, exposure to cold causes urticaria and angioedema either during exposure or after rewarming (cold urticaria).

Understanding allergic asthma

Allergy may cause two types of asthma: extrinsic asthma and allergic bronchopulmonary aspergillosis (ABPA). Assessing any potentially asthmatic patient demands a careful search for allergies. You can suspect a link with allergy when an asthmatic patient has:
- a family history of allergic diseases
- seasonal exacerbation of symptoms
- concomitant allergic rhinitis or other allergic disease
- slightly to moderately elevated serum eosinophil count (300 to 1,000/mm^3)
- elevated sputum eosinophil count
- symptom onset before age 40. Allergic asthma accounts for less than half of all asthma cases after age 40. Before age 30, it accounts for about 90%.

Several diagnostic studies can help confirm allergic asthma. *Skin tests* confirm an IgE response to a suspected allergen, but they can't establish a cause-and-effect relationship. *Serum IgE levels* can be useful because about 60% of allergic asthmatics have levels above 300 ng/ml. However, because 40% of patients have a normal IgE level, the test can't confirm a diagnosis. The *bronchial provocation test* has positive results in patients who have positive skin tests.

In ABPA, one of five pulmonary diseases caused by *Aspergillus*, a subacute inflammatory reaction occurs when IgE and IgG antibodies respond to growth of this fungus in the respiratory tree. Suspect ABPA in asthmatic patients with:
- an eosinophil count above 10,000/mm^3
- positive immediate or late-phase (or Arthus) reaction to skin test for *Aspergillus* antigen
- IgG antibodies to *Aspergillus* antigens
- presence of *Aspergillus* in sputum
- elevated IgE levels
- pulmonary infiltrates, often transitory
- central, saccular bronchiectasis
- expectorated brown plugs or specks.

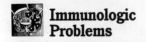

Hypersensitivity Disorders

Atopic dermatitis: Caused by allergy?

Could atopic dermatitis be a cutaneous form of atopic hypersensitivity? Some researchers think so, based on two facts. First, atopic dermatitis is often associated with allergic rhinitis and asthma in affected patients and among members of the same family. Second, affected patients usually demonstrate extremely high serum IgE levels.

Despite these facts, it's tough to prove a link between atopic dermatitis and hypersensitivity. That's because some studies suggest that atopic dermatitis could be a skin abnormality of metabolic or biochemical origin, perhaps with genetic ties to elevated IgE levels. Other studies also imply a partial T-cell deficiency. What's more, the severity of atopic dermatitis doesn't usually correlate with the patient's exposure to known allergens. And atopic dermatitis doesn't respond to immunotherapy.

Typically, atopic dermatitis arises at age 3 to 6 months but may appear first in childhood, adolescence, or occasionally in adult life. When assessing a patient for atopic dermatitis, look for:
- dry skin and pruritus
- characteristic features of eczema, produced by chronic scratching and rubbing
- lesions on the forehead, cheeks, and extensor surfaces of infants' extremities
- lesions distributed in a flexural pattern, with predilection for the antecubital and popliteal areas and the neck
- lesions on the face, especially around the eyes and ears.

Initially, active lesions are erythematous and pruritic. Scratching will produce excoriations, papules, and scaling. Treated promptly, the skin will revert to normal; however, prolonged scratching will cause lichenified skin and altered pigmentation.

Treatment includes meticulous skin care, environmental control, drugs, and avoidance of allergens, as indicated. Soothing topical lubricants moisten the skin, making it less itchy. Topical corticosteroids or even a brief course of systemic corticosteroids may be used. Oral antihistamines can help control pruritus. The disease often improves spontaneously during summer months.

- Exercise, overheating, or emotional stress can cause small wheals with a large area of surrounding flare.
- Emotional trauma may provoke acute urticaria or angioedema or aggravate the chronic form of the disease.

Your assessment should also rule out an underlying local or systemic infection, which may provoke urticaria. Parasitic infection often elevates the eosinophil count and serum IgE. Prodromal phases of hepatitis B, infectious mononucleosis, and other viral infections commonly cause urticaria. However, bacterial infections rarely cause urticaria.

Assess for systemic disorders, too. Urticaria has been linked to such neoplasms as Hodgkin's disease and lymphomas, and to such connective tissue disorders as SLE.

Intervention. If foods or drugs are the culprit, advise the patient to avoid the allergen. If environmental factors are the cause, advise him to avoid heat, sunlight, or cold. If infection is implicated, encourage treatment. Also expect the doctor to order antihistamines. Epinephrine injections may relieve urticaria briefly as well as treat pharyngeal or laryngeal edema.

Hereditary angioedema

This rare, autosomal dominant form of angioedema results from a deficiency of C1 inactivator. This deficiency causes uncontrolled activation of early components of the complement system. A kinin-like substance generated in the plasma induces recurrent episodes of angioedema in the GI tract, genitourinary tract, and larynx.

Assessment. Diagnosis of a complement deficiency is difficult and requires careful interpretation of both clinical features and laboratory results. Clinical effects usually arise during childhood with recurrent episodes of subcutaneous or submucosal edema at irregular intervals of weeks, months, or years, often following trauma or stress. Symptoms may include swelling in the face, hands, abdomen, or throat. GI involvement may cause nausea, vomiting, and severe abdominal pain. Laryngeal angioedema may cause fatal airway obstruction. Urticaria doesn't occur.

Intervention. To prevent or ameliorate attacks, the doctor may order such plasma inhibitors as aminocaproic acid. Taken orally, these drugs achieve their effects possibly by inhibiting fibrinolytic generation of the active kinin peptide. Androgen therapy using methyltestosterone or attenuated sex hormones such as oxymetholone and danazol may prevent attacks. These hormones also significantly increase C1 inactivator and C4 serum levels, and may possibly correct the inherited deficiency.

Sarcoidosis

This multisystem, granulomatous disorder occurs most commonly in young adults, often with the greatest frequency and severity among blacks. Although the lung is most commonly involved, sarcoidosis can affect any organ of the body.

The cause of sarcoidosis is unknown. However, inflammatory cells—primarily monocytes, macrophages, and T cells—accumulate in involved tissues and form granulomas. An increased number of B cells and plasma cells also occur in the affected tissues.

Continued on page 66

Hypersensitivity Disorders

Hemolytic disease of the newborn

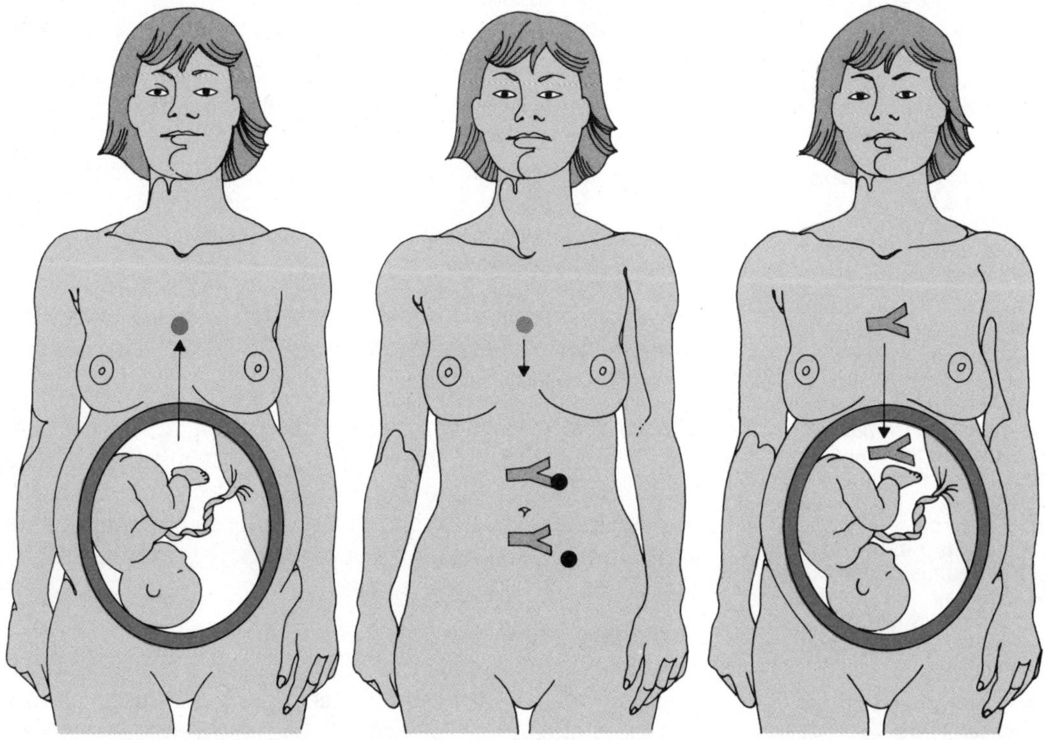

This Type II hypersensitivity disorder occurs in newborn infants when a pregnant woman has been sensitized to blood group antigens on her infant's erythrocytes. Her immune system then produces IgG antibodies to these antigens that cross the placenta and destroy fetal red blood cells.

This condition most commonly involves the Rhesus D (RhD) antigen. Consider, for instance, an Rh^- mother carrying an Rh^+ infant. The Rh^- mother becomes sensitized to the Rh^+ red cells, usually during birth, when her immune system recognizes fetal red cells that leak from the placenta into her bloodstream. This stimulates production of IgG anti-Rh antibodies. In subsequent pregnancies, the mother becomes repeatedly immunized, placing the second and later infants at an increased risk for hemolytic disease.

To prevent this reaction, administer anti-RhD antibodies (RhoGam, for example) to the mother immediately after delivery of an Rh^+ baby, thereby eliminating the Rh^+ red cells and preventing sensitization.

Selected hypersensitivity disorders—*continued*

Assessment. The combination of fever, erythema nodosum, iritis, and polyarthritis strongly suggests acute sarcoidosis. The patient may describe an insidious onset of fatigue, weight loss, malaise, weakness, anorexia, fever, sweats, a nonproductive cough, and progressive exertional dyspnea.

More than 90% of patients show pulmonary symptoms. Pulmonary function studies may reveal such evidence of restrictive lung disease as reduced lung volume, decreased diffusion capacity, and exercise-induced hypoxemia. Patients with advanced disease may also show evidence of an obstructive ventilatory defect. However, normal pulmonary function results don't rule out sarcoidosis.

Routine chest X-rays can detect many asymptomatic patients. When studying chest X-rays, doctors look for the following abnormalities:

- *Type 0 involvement*—no abnormalities
- *Type I involvement*—bilateral hilar adenopathy alone

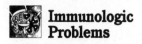

Hypersensitivity Disorders

• *Type II involvement*—hilar adenopathy and parenchymal abnormalities
• *Type III involvement*—parenchymal abnormalities without hilar adenopathy.

Other evidence that suggests sarcoidosis includes:
• T lymphocytopenia
• anergy to various skin tests
• hypergammaglobulinemia
• circulating immune complexes
• increased serum angiotensin-converting enzyme activity
• increased macrophages and T-helper cells in bronchoalveolar lavage fluid.

A firm diagnosis requires three elements: a compatible clinical picture, histologic evidence of systemic granulomatous disease, and absence of exposure to any other agent known to cause granulomatous disease.

Intervention. Treatment includes symptomatic and supportive care as well as drug therapy. If the patient experiences progressive loss of lung function, cardiac disease, granulomatous uveitis, or central nervous system disease, expect the doctor to order corticosteroid therapy for as long as the disease is active. He may also order corticosteroids to relieve such associated symptoms as joint involvement and erythema nodosum.

Self-Test

1. In systemic lupus erythematosus (SLE), the antinuclear antibody titer is normally:
a. high **b.** low **c.** normal

2. Treatment for SLE may include all of the following except:
a. beta blockers **b.** antimalarials **c.** corticosteroids **d.** nonsteroidal anti-inflammatory drugs

3. Sjögren's syndrome is characterized by:
a. dry eyes caused by reduced lacrimal secretions **b.** dry mouth caused by reduced salivary secretions **c.** both a and b **d.** none of the above

4. T cells and macrophages primarily mediate:
a. Type I hypersensitivity reactions **b.** Type II hypersensitivity reactions **c.** Type III hypersensitivity reactions **d.** Type IV hypersensitivity reactions

5. The major chemical mediator of anaphylaxis is:
a. slow-reacting substance of anaphylaxis **b.** eosinophil chemotactic factor of anaphylaxis **c.** histamine **d.** serotonin

6. In an allergic patient, you can expect the eosinophil count to:
a. increase **b.** decrease **c.** stay within the normal range

7. When treating a patient with anaphylaxis, expect to administer:
a. aminophylline **b.** epinephrine **c.** diphenhydramine **d.** cimetidine

Answers (page number shows where answer appears in text)
1. **a** (page 27) 2. **a** (page 31) 3. **c** (page 37) 4. **d** (page 46) 5. **c** (page 48) 6. **a** (page 55) 7. **b** (page 61)

Acquired Immunodeficiency Syndrome: Nursing Challenge

Mary Ann Colletti, RN, MS, wrote the section of this chapter dealing with adult AIDS. Ms. Colletti is an AIDS clinical nurse specialist at Rush-Presbyterian-St. Luke's Medical Center in Chicago. **Laura S. Bradford, BSN, PhD,** wrote the material on pediatric AIDS. Dr. Bradford is a level D staff nurse in the special care nursery of the same medical center.

An immunodeficiency of epidemic proportions, acquired immunodeficiency syndrome (AIDS) is one of the most serious health challenges of our time. AIDS is characterized by chronic wasting syndrome, dementia, opportunistic infection (notably *Pneumocystis carinii* pneumonia), or malignancy (notably Kaposi's sarcoma)—or by some combination of these conditions. AIDS apparently results from infection with human immunodeficiency virus (HIV).

What is HIV and how does it lead to AIDS? How should you care for an AIDS patient? What measures should you take to prevent transmission of this deadly disease? Knowing the answers to these questions will help you give better, more confident nursing care. In this chapter, we'll discuss these topics and others, including the pathophysiology and epidemiology of AIDS, the opportunistic infections and malignancies that affect AIDS patients, assessment measures and findings, interventions, and the special needs of children with AIDS.

What is HIV?

One of several human retroviruses, HIV has been called by several names: lymphadenopathy-associated virus (LAV), human T-cell lymphotropic virus type III (HTLV-III), and AIDS-associated retrovirus (ARV). (See *Human retroviruses: The name game.*) Retroviruses contain the enzyme reverse transcriptase, which makes a deoxyribonucleic acid (DNA) copy of ribonucleic acid (RNA). DNA, in turn, integrates with host cell DNA.

HIV can replicate in a limited number of cells in the human body, including lymphocytes, macrophages, and central nervous system (CNS) cells. Like other viruses, HIV is parasitic: it survives only in living host cells, dying quickly once outside the body. It cannot survive on inanimate surfaces. Also like other retroviruses, the HIV genome integrates into the host cell genome, producing progeny viruses. After infection, antibodies develop to several HIV proteins, but these antibodies don't necessarily protect the patient. HIV has a remarkable ability to induce a persistent viremic (carrier) state in infected patients despite the presence of antibodies.

HIV consists of an RNA core surrounded by a protein shell and a lipoprotein envelope. This surface envelope contains several glycoprotein molecules; at least one of them (gp 120) attaches to a receptor on certain cells in the host's immune system. However, molecules on HIV's surface vary depending on the viral strain, making HIV quite versatile. (See *What happens in HIV infection*, page 70.)

Recently, a second virus that appears to be an HIV mutation was isolated. Called HIV-2, this virus causes symptoms similar to those produced by HIV infection.

After exposure to HIV, the patient develops an antibody response, usually in 6 to 12 weeks but occasionally only after 6 months. Detection of serum HIV antibodies indicates exposure to the virus and the potential for developing AIDS and transmitting the virus to others.

HIV's long incubation period sets it apart from other viruses. After infection, symptoms may not develop in adults for 6 months to 7 years or more (some studies indicate up to 15 years). Once infected,

NF-kappa B: An HIV trigger?

Can bacterial, viral, or protozoal infections activate a dormant HIV infection? Researchers think so, now that they've identified a protein unique to activated T cells. The protein, NF-kappa B, greatly heightens in vitro expression of HIV.

Researchers already knew that HIV established itself better in activated T cells than in resting T cells. So they looked for a factor unique to these activated cells. First, they isolated the HIV viral enhancer/promoter region that acts as an on-off switch after the virus merges with the host genome. Next, they found that the protein NF-kappa B binds to this region and induces transcription of HIV DNA in T cells; this protein appears only in activated cells. Since this HIV-enhancing protein appears during viral infection, researchers now believe that concurrent viral infections could trigger HIV expression.

Although this research was done in vitro, it provides yet another reason for HIV-infected patients to reduce their exposure to infection.

Acquired Immunodeficiency Syndrome

Human retroviruses: The name game

News about human immunodeficiency virus (HIV) changes almost daily. So, it seems, has the terminology associated with the virus. Below are the names currently used to describe five types of the retrovirus human T-cell leukemia-lymphoma virus (HTLV).

HTLV-I, a T-cell leukemia–associated virus, causes adult T-cell leukemia-lymphoma, a cancer that attacks blood and bone marrow cells. Transmission occurs through sexual activity and sharing of infected needles, leading experts to believe that this virus is related to acquired immunodeficiency syndrome (AIDS).

HTLV-II is also a T-cell leukemia–associated virus.

HTLV-III, the first to be called the AIDS virus, is an immunodeficiency-associated virus. Once called lymphadenopathy-associated virus (LAV), HTLV-III is now known as human immunodeficiency virus (HIV) or HIV-1.

HTLV-IV is an immunodeficiency-associated virus known to cause AIDS. Once called LAV-2, this virus is now known as HIV-2. Although HIV-2 differs genetically from HIV-1, it attacks the body in similar ways and causes the same effects as HIV-1.

HTLV-V, recently discovered in a patient with cutaneous T-cell lymphoma, is a human retrovirus associated with greater immunosuppression than HTLV-I but less than HIV-1.

patients probably harbor the virus for the rest of their lives. Although no one knows how many infected patients go on to develop AIDS, some researchers estimate the likelihood to be two out of three. What's more, concurrent infection with other organisms, use of psychoactive drugs, stress, and malnutrition may contribute to development of AIDS.

HIV transmission

HIV has been isolated from blood, semen, vaginal secretions, breast milk, saliva, tears, urine, cerebrospinal fluid (CSF), and alveolar fluid. However, only blood and semen are known to transmit the virus, although vaginal secretions and breast milk may transmit it as well. Isolation of the virus from a body fluid doesn't necessarily mean that the fluid acts as a route of transmission.

HIV has also been isolated from brain tissue, especially glial cells. This discovery means that the CNS, which is protected by the blood-brain barrier, might serve as a haven for the virus. It also means that any drugs used to treat AIDS must cross the blood-brain barrier to be effective.

HIV transmission can occur in three ways: through exposure to infected blood (possibly via transfusion, I.V. drug use, or accidental parenteral inoculation), through sexual activity with an infected person, or perinatally to an infant from an infected mother. (See *How HIV is transmitted*, page 70.)

Transfusion. HIV has been transmitted through whole blood, blood components, plasma, and clotting factors. No other blood products (such as immunoglobulin, albumin, plasma protein fraction, or hepatitis B vaccine) have been implicated.

Screening of donated blood and plasma for HIV antibodies began in April, 1985. This screening program, along with heat treatment of clotting factor concentrates and donor screening, has dramatically reduced the risk of HIV exposure through transfusion. However, a majority of the hemophiliacs in the United States have already been infected with HIV; an estimated 12,000 people in this country acquired the virus from transfusions before screening began.

I.V. drug use. I.V. drug users play a key role in transmitting the HIV virus because they're the main bridge to other adults through heterosexual contact, and to children through perinatal transmission. Heterosexual I.V. drug users most commonly become infected with HIV by sharing needles and other drug apparatus with people already infected.

Parenteral inoculation. This transmission route depends in large part on the amount of inoculum on the needle. Because the amount of inoculum on the tip of a needle is quite small, the risk of a health care worker becoming infected in this way is very low, especially if the worker follows precautions recommended by the Centers for Disease Control (CDC). These precautions are discussed later in the chapter.

Sexual contact. HIV can be transmitted through homosexual or heterosexual contact with an infected person. The virus may be transmitted in semen or may enter the blood through breaks in mucous membranes. No one knows the risk of acquiring HIV infection from single or multiple sexual encounters with an infected

Continued on page 71

Acquired Immunodeficiency Syndrome

How HIV is transmitted

The human immunodeficiency virus (HIV), only slightly more than 100 nm in diameter, can be transmitted in the following ways:

Blood transmission
- Transfusion of contaminated blood or blood products
- Sharing of contaminated needles and accidental needlesticks
- Exposure through open wounds or mucous membranes

Sexual transmission
- Homosexual, between men
- Heterosexual (either partner can infect the other)

Perinatal transmission
- Intrauterine exposure
- Peripartum exposure

HIV can't be transmitted by insect stings or bites, close personal contact between household members, or health-care procedures that don't involve exposure to blood.

What happens in HIV infection

In acquired immunodeficiency syndrome (AIDS), the number of T4 (T-helper) cells declines, mainly because human immunodeficiency virus (HIV) selectively binds with and destroys them. The main glycoprotein in HIV's lipid envelope, a substance called gp 120, binds HIV to T4 receptor sites.

After binding to a target cell, HIV enters the cell and sheds its envelope. Just how the virus enters the cell isn't yet known, but its mechanism may be similar to receptor-mediated endocytosis. Or the HIV envelope might fuse directly with the cell membrane, mediating entry into the membrane. Once HIV enters the cell, the enzyme reverse transcriptase transcribes the genomic RNA into DNA. Afterward, during cell division, the DNA is circularized and integrated into the host genome by a virus-encoded enzyme. At this point, HIV's replication cycle may be suspended until the infected T4 cell becomes activated.

T4 cells can be activated by such pathogens as cytomegalovirus, Epstein-Barr virus, hepatitis A and B virus, and herpes simplex virus, especially type 2. They can also be stimulated allogeneically by exposure to such body fluids as semen or blood. Activation is followed by transcription, protein synthesis with post-translational processing (protein cleavage and glycosylation), and assembling of viral proteins and genomic RNA at the cell surface, where mature viral particles (virions) bud and break free of the cell. HIV reproduction kills T4 cells, although no one knows exactly how.

Because T4 cells are critically important in the immune response, destruction of even part of their population can cause immunodeficiencies. These immunodeficiencies leave the patient vulnerable to the potentially fatal opportunistic infections and malignancies characteristic of AIDS.

HIV replication cycle

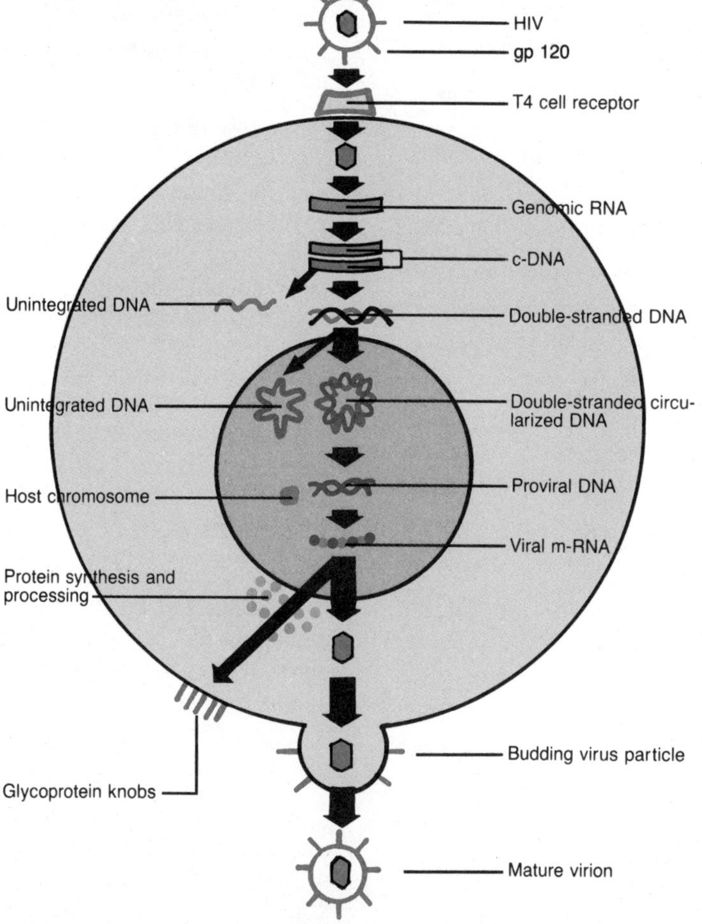

Acquired Immunodeficiency Syndrome

New theories on AIDS pathophysiology

Researchers continue to learn about human immunodeficiency virus (HIV) and how it relates to acquired immunodeficiency syndrome (AIDS). Some recent studies suggest that macrophages may play a larger role in AIDS than previously thought. In fact, some researchers think that AIDS may be more of a macrophage disease than a T-cell disease. This may help to explain why AIDS has such a long latency period and why the virus seems to escape immune detection.

Infected macrophages seem to act as reservoirs for HIV, perhaps transporting the virus to and from various parts of the body. HIV-infected macrophages may also prevent T-cell activation. Diagnostic tests that detect the virus in macrophages (such as the Cetus test) are now being developed for commercial use.

Based on another controversial study, University of California molecular biologist Peter Duesberg questions whether HIV even causes AIDS. After studying HIV and other retroviruses, Duesberg doubts that HIV—as a T-cell infection—could cause AIDS on its own. Additional study should shed light on this theory.

Continued

person. Researchers still haven't found a clear connection between seropositivity, the number of sexual encounters, the length of the relationship, and specific sexual practices (except for receptive anal intercourse, which is a major route of transmission). Biological factors, such as susceptibility and differing infectability among viral strains, may be important determinants.

Perinatal transmission. Most infants and small children infected with HIV acquire the virus from their infected mothers in utero, during delivery, or shortly after birth. Two routes of infection have been documented: to the fetus through the maternal circulation, and to the infant through inoculation or ingestion of blood or other infected fluids. A third route—to the infant through infected breast milk—is theoretically possible, although it hasn't been documented yet.

Pathophysiology

To understand why and how clinical manifestations of HIV infection occur, you must first understand how HIV affects the immune system and how AIDS may later develop. To start, we'll briefly review immune system components and their functions. For more details, refer back to Chapter 1.

The immune system has two primary types of cells:

- lymphoid cells or lymphocytes, including B cells and T cells
- nonlymphoid cells, including platelets, red blood cells, and phagocytic cells. Phagocytic cells include granulocytes and monocytes (or macrophages). Neutrophils, the most common granulocyte, provide the body's main defense against bacteria and other extracellular pathogens; HIV doesn't seem to infect them. Macrophages are derived from white cells called monocytes. Unlike neutrophils, which remain in the circulation and enter the tissues only when the body responds to pathogenic invasion, macrophages differentiate into active and aggressive cells within host tissues. Like neutrophils, they phagocytize and kill foreign substances. Recent studies show that HIV does infect macrophages. These studies have demonstrated HIV's presence not only in T cells, but also in macrophages and other white blood cells that may harbor the virus, produce more virus, and perhaps transmit the disease. This may cause a breakdown between macrophages and lymphocytes, affecting the immune system's ability to destroy the virus.

Lymphocytes help defend the body against fungi, viruses, protozoa, and certain intracellular bacteria—organisms that aren't handled as efficiently as simple bacteria. They're divided into two types: B cells and T cells. B cells differentiate into plasma cells and secrete antibodies in response to such foreign substances as microbial pathogens. B-cell immune responses are called *humoral immunity*.

T cells consist of many different groups of cells that become activated during infections with fungi, protozoa, viruses, and intracellular bacteria. T-cell immune responses are called *cell-mediated immunity*. Two T-cell groups come into play in HIV infection: T-helper cells (also called T4 cells) and T-suppressor cells (also called T8 cells). T-suppressor cells inhibit the immune response, whereas T-helper cells enhance it.

Continued on page 72

Acquired Immunodeficiency Syndrome

Continued

HIV has an affinity for T-helper cells. Once inside the cell, the virus merges with the cell's genome and then replicates within the cell. When HIV is released from the T-helper cell, the cell is destroyed. HIV then moves to other T-helper cells and replicates again, resulting in widespread destruction and reduced numbers of T-helper cells. Normally, T cells number about 1,150 to 1,550/mm^3, with T-helper cells making up 27% to 55% and T-suppressor cells making up 13% to 23%. In a normally functioning immune system, the ratio of T-helper cells to T-suppressor cells ranges from 1.3 to 2.9. But in an HIV-infected person, the loss of T-helper cells reverses this ratio and T-suppressor cells predominate. Because T-helper cells prompt the immune system to combat fungi, protozoa, viruses, and certain intracellular bacteria, their destruction leaves the body vulnerable to opportunistic infections with these organisms and to certain neoplasms. (See *Opportunistic infections commonly associated with AIDS.*) Besides the HIV infection itself, most patients with AIDS develop opportunistic infections or malignancies.

Opportunistic infections. Infections that develop in AIDS patients are called opportunistic because the pathogens take advantage of the suppressed immune system, specifically the T cell–mediated response. The pathogens involved appear frequently in immunosuppressed patients. Many opportunistic infections are complicated and disseminated, so they tend to resist treatment or recur in spite of conventional therapy. Their type, location, and severity usually reflect the extent of immunosuppression.

Fungal infections. These may include candidiasis, which may involve the esophagus, trachea, bronchi, or lungs; extrapulmonary cryptococcosis, which often involves the brain; and histoplasmosis, which may disseminate beyond the lungs or lymph nodes.

Viral infections. These include cytomegalovirus (CMV) infection in organs other than the liver, spleen, or lymph nodes in a patient older than 1 month; herpes simplex causing mucocutaneous ulcers persisting longer than 1 month; and bronchitis, pneumonitis, or esophagitis in a patient older than 1 month. Progressive multifocal leukoencephalopathy caused by papovavirus may also occur.

Protozoal infections. Besides *Pneumocystis carinii* pneumonia (PCP) (see sidebar), protozoal infections include *Cryptosporidium*, *Isospora belli*, and *Toxoplasma gondii* (associated with cerebral abscess in patients older than 1 month). These infections may cause chronic, voluminous diarrhea leading to severe malabsorption, malnutrition, electrolyte deficits, and other complications that don't respond well to conventional treatments.

Bacterial infections. These usually involve such intracellular pathogens as *Salmonella* and *Mycobacterium tuberculosis,* which affect organs beyond the lung. Other infectious organisms include *M. avium-intracellularis* and *M. kansasii*, which affect sites other than or in addition to the lungs, skin, or cervical or hilar lymph nodes. Most bacterial infections result from neutropenia, a common adverse effect of many AIDS drug therapies.

Pneumocystis carinii pneumonia

The most common opportunistic infection associated with AIDS, *Pneumocystis carinii* pneumonia (PCP) accounts for up to 80% of all opportunistic infections in AIDS. Although PCP can occur with other immunologic disorders, it doesn't respond as well to treatment and causes more relapses in patients with AIDS. Patients also suffer a high incidence of adverse effects from trimethoprim-sulfamethoxazole (TMP-SMX), the drug used most often to treat PCP.

Pneumocystis carinii, the causative organism, is a ubiquitous, one-celled protozoan. Although it doesn't infect healthy people, it can infect the pulmonary tissues of immunosuppressed people. Numerous cysts composed of clumped organisms multiply in alveolar spaces and eventually cause obstructive disease.

Signs and symptoms of PCP range from mild fever and dyspnea on exertion to respiratory failure. Successful management hinges on early detection of pulmonary involvement.

Confirming diagnosis of PCP requires all of the following:

- dyspnea on exertion or nonproductive cough within the past 3 months
- chest X-ray showing diffuse bilateral interstitial infiltrates, or a gallium scan showing diffuse bilateral pulmonary disease
- a PaO_2 of 70 mm Hg or less, a low respiratory diffusing capacity (<80% of predicted values), or an increase in the alveolar-arterial oxygen tension gradient
- no signs of bacterial pneumonia.

Supportive care includes bed rest and oxygen. Drugs of choice for treating PCP in AIDS patients include TMP-SMX and pentamidine isethionate. Trimetrexate has also been used. Investigational drugs include dapsone-trimethoprim, sulfadoxine-pyrimethamine, and difluromethylornithane. Corticosteroids have been used in acute stages to reduce lung inflammation.

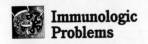

Acquired Immunodeficiency Syndrome

Malignancies. Also considered to be opportunistic diseases, malignancies occur because the T cell–mediated response fails to thwart the growth of malignant cells. Malignancies occur less commonly than opportunistic infections in AIDS patients; Kaposi's sarcoma occurs the most frequently. (See *Kaposi's sarcoma*, page 75.)

Primary brain lymphoma, also common among AIDS patients, causes changes in mental status. Although the tumor can be treated

Continued on page 74

Opportunistic infections commonly associated with AIDS

Infection	Affected areas	Treatment
VIRUSES		
Cytomegalovirus (CMV)	• Lungs: pneumonia • GI tract: diarrhea, colitis • Liver: elevated liver enzymes • Retina: large hemorrhages, white exudates, visual changes leading to blindness • Lymphocytes: positive antibody titers • Brain: encephalitis	• Acyclovir • Ganciclovir (also known as DHPG): experimental for CMV retinitis
Herpes simplex	• Perineal, perianal, and scrotal areas; face; esophagus; colon: mucocutaneous ulcers lasting longer than 1 month	• Acyclovir, vidarabine, fluoroidoaracytosine (also known as FIAC)
Herpes zoster	• Disseminated: weeping, raised, coalesced, pruritic rash, usually on buttocks, back, and legs	•Acyclovir, vidarabine, FIAC
FUNGI		
Candida albicans	• Mouth, esophagus: difficult, painful swallowing; white coating or plaque in oral mucosa • Anus: white coating or plaque in rectal mucosa • Axilla, groin, systemic: skin lesions	• Miconazole, nystatin, clotrimazole, mycelex, ketoconazole, I.V. amphotericin B, 5-flucytosine
Cryptococcus neoformans	• Brain: meningitis • Blood: fungicemia	• Amphotericin B, 5-flucytosine, ketoconazole
PROTOZOA		
Pneumocystis carinii	• Disseminated: initially, diarrhea, night sweats, fever, weight loss, unexplained lymphodenopathy; later, dyspnea, dry cough, tachypnea, cyanosis, diffuse crackles, severe hypoxemia • Retina: cotton-wool exudates	• Trimethoprim-sulfamethoxazole (also known as TMP-SMX) • Pentamidine • Trimetrexate with leucovorin • Experimental: dapsone-trimethoprim; sulfadoxine-pyrimethamine; dapsone; BW301; difluromethylornithane (also known as DFMO)
Toxoplasma gondii	• Brain: abscess, diffuse encephalopathy, meningoencephalitis	• Sulfadiazine and pyrimethamine with leucovorin
Cryptosporidium	• GI tract: soft stools to severe diarrhea	• No effective treatment known • Possible spiramycin or combined quinine and clindamycin • opiate-based antidiarrheal drugs • I.V. hyperalimentation, fluid replacements
MYCOBACTERIA		
Mycobacterium avium and tuberculosis	• Lungs: chronic cough, hemoptysis • Liver, spleen, lymph nodes, bone marrow: fatigue, weakness, weight loss, fever	• Usually a combination of two or more of the following: rifampin, isoniazid, ethambutol, ethionamide, streptomycin, capreomycin, cycloserine, pyrazinamide • Experimental: ansamycin, clofazamine

Acquired Immunodeficiency Syndrome

Continued

with radiation, prognosis is poor. Prognosis is also poor for other non-Hodgkin's lymphomas (such as high-grade B-cell non-Hodgkin's lymphoma) because they tend to be poorly differentiated. Lymphocytic leukemia, rapidly progressive Hodgkin's disease, solid tumors, and multiple myeloma have also been reported among AIDS patients.

Epidemiology

AIDS is the only manifestation of HIV infection that must be reported to the CDC. Since AIDS was first recognized as a communicable disease, the CDC definition has changed several times. In August 1987, the definition was expanded to include signs of profound immunosuppression, such as severe wasting syndrome and progressive dementia. (See *How the CDC defines AIDS*, page 76.)

The number of reported AIDS cases reflects only a small percentage of the people who are actually infected with HIV. Those who have positive antibody tests or AIDS-related complex (ARC) aren't reported to the CDC, so they're not included in national statistics. Some researchers estimate that for every reported case of AIDS, 50 to 75 people carry the virus. The expanded CDC definition may provide a more accurate estimate of how many people are infected with HIV.

No one knows precisely where HIV originated or how it entered the United States. However, its pattern of worldwide transmission suggests that the virus originated in central Africa and spread first to the Caribbean (especially Haiti) and then to North America, Australia, Europe, and Asia. The retrovirus may have originated in primates and then spread to humans and mutated. Studies show that African green monkeys develop an AIDS-like illness after infection with the simian form of HIV.

The World Health Organization (WHO) estimates that 100,000 to 150,000 people have AIDS worldwide, and that 5 million to 10 million people carry HIV. In the next 5 years, WHO estimates that 500,000 to 3 million new AIDS cases will arise from those people infected now. The CDC estimates that 1 million to 1.5 million Americans now carry the virus, and that 20% to 30% of them will develop AIDS by the end of 1991.

Research shows that HIV-infected patients develop AIDS at a variable rate, making predictions difficult. Apparently, AIDS develops more commonly 5 to 10 years after HIV infection than during the first 5 years. Specifically, about 20% to 30% of infected patients develop AIDS during the first 5 years, after which the rate appears to accelerate. About 75% show some signs of illness 7 years after infection; up to 36% of infected patients go on to develop AIDS at that point. Researchers still don't know how many patients infected with HIV develop AIDS. Predictions range from 65% to 100% over a 16-year period.

Although the infections and diseases that characterize AIDS are ultimately fatal, life expectancy varies. Most patients die within 2 years of diagnosis, and up to 98% die within 3 years of diagnosis.

75 Immunodeficiency Disorders

Acquired Immunodeficiency Syndrome

Kaposi's sarcoma

The most common malignancy in patients with AIDS, Kaposi's sarcoma affects endothelial tissue, which compromises all blood vessels. Once seen only in elderly men of Mediterranean descent, this malignancy was first linked to AIDS in 1981.

In its original form, Kaposi's sarcoma affects the cutaneous tissues, usually of the legs. It can exist for a decade or longer without harming the internal organs. The AIDS-associated form, a far more aggressive disease, invades the deeper organs and tissues, especially of the GI tract. It produces small, multicentric lesions over the entire body. Cherry red or purple, these lesions may be slightly raised. They may also be isolated or follow a linear pattern. In advanced stages, the disease obstructs the lymphatic system, causing leg, head, and neck edema.

Kaposi's sarcoma is diagnosed by biopsy. Its treatment varies, depending on whether the disease is restricted to the skin or involves the deeper tissues. Cutaneous lesions are treated for cosmetic reasons with electron beam therapy. Chemotherapy is the treatment of choice for deeper lesions, although they may also be irradiated. Kaposi's sarcoma carries a better prognosis than *Pneumocystis carinii* pneumonia and other opportunistic infections associated with AIDS.

The chart at right shows treatments for various signs and symptoms of Kaposi's sarcoma.

Signs and symptoms	Treatments
Minimal Kaposi's sarcoma: No fever, infections, night sweats, or weight loss	• Experimental immunomodulators, antiviral drugs, or both • Vinblastine alternating with vincristine; other single-agent chemotherapy
Minimal Kaposi's sarcoma: History of infections, fever, or both; night sweats; or weight loss	• Vinblastine alternating with vincristine; other single-agent chemotherapy • Experimental drugs
Advanced cutaneous, rapidly progressing, or pulmonary Kaposi's sarcoma	• Etoposide; low-dose doxorubicin; other single-agent chemotherapy • Experimental drugs
Kaposi's sarcoma with neutropenia or thrombocytopenia	• Vincristine or bleomycin
Painful, bulky Kaposi's sarcoma or lymphedema	• Radiation therapy

All U.S. states, the District of Columbia, and the four U.S. territories have reported cases of AIDS. New York, New Jersey, California, Texas, and Florida head the list. The ten cities with the most AIDS cases, in descending order, are New York City; San Francisco; Los Angeles; Houston; Washington, D.C.; Newark; Miami; Chicago; Dallas; and Philadelphia.

Almost half the AIDS patients in the U.S. are between age 30 and 39. So far, a higher percentage of Blacks and Hispanics are affected than Caucasians, although the actual number is smaller. About two thirds of all AIDS patients are homosexual or bisexual men, making this the largest risk group in the U.S. But the infection rate among homosexuals appears to be declining because of safer sex practices. Bisexual men continue to serve as a bridge of infection between the homosexual community and the general population. In addition, about 17% of adults with AIDS are I.V. drug users, who also may spread the disease through heterosexual activity. Homosexual or bisexual men who also use I.V. drugs comprise about 7% of the adult AIDS population.

Heterosexuals account for about 4% of all AIDS patients. Included in this group are men and women who've had sexual contact with a person who carries HIV or who has AIDS, as well as people outside known risk groups but who were born in countries—such as African countries—where heterosexual transmission of the virus is common. Over the past few years, the number of heterosexuals with AIDS has increased. Although infection can occur as a result of a single, unprotected sexual encounter, women are probably more likely to contract HIV infection from men than vice versa.

So far, more heterosexual women than heterosexual men have AIDS; this is the only transmission category where women outnumber

Continued on page 77

Acquired Immunodeficiency Syndrome

How the CDC defines AIDS

In August 1987, the Centers for Disease Control (CDC) revised the case definition of acquired immunodeficiency syndrome (AIDS) to streamline and improve the accuracy of disease reporting nationwide. According to the revised definition, AIDS is an illness characterized by one or more indicator diseases and based on laboratory evidence of human immunodeficiency virus (HIV) infection. Details of the CDC's revised definition appear below.

Without laboratory evidence of HIV infection

If laboratory tests for HIV infection weren't performed or prove inconclusive, and if a patient has none of the causes of immunodeficiency listed in Group A, then the patient can be considered to have AIDS if he has a *definitive diagnosis* of any one of the disorders listed in Group B.

Group A
- Systemic corticosteroid or other immunosuppressive/cytotoxic therapy 3 months or less before the start of a Group B disease
- Any of the following diseases diagnosed within 3 months of diagnosing a Group B disease: Hodgkin's disease, non-Hodgkin's lymphoma (other than primary brain lymphoma), lymphocytic leukemia, multiple myeloma, any other cancer of lymphoreticular or histiocytic tissue, or angioimmunoblastic lymphadenopathy
- A congenital immunodeficiency syndrome atypical of HIV infection (hypogammaglobulinemia, for example)

Group B
- Bronchitis, pneumonitis, or esophagitis persisting longer than 1 month
- Candidiasis of the esophagus, trachea, bronchi, or lungs
- Cryptosporidiosis accompanied by diarrhea that persists longer than 1 month
- Cytomegalovirus infection in an organ other than the liver, spleen, or lymph nodes in a patient more than 1 month old
- Extrapulmonary cryptococcosis
- Herpes simplex ulcers persisting longer than 1 month
- Kaposi's sarcoma in a patient under 60 years
- Lymphoid interstitial pneumonia, pulmonary lymphoid hyperplasia, or both in a child under 13 years
- *Mycobacterium avium* complex or *M. kansasii* infection at a site other than or in addition to the lungs, skin, or cervical or hilar lymph nodes
- *Pneumocystis carinii* pneumonia (PCP)
- Primary brain lymphoma in a patient under 60 years
- Progressive multifocal leukoencephalopathy
- Toxoplasmosis of the brain affecting a patient less than 1 month old.

With laboratory evidence of HIV infection

Regardless of the other causes of immunodeficiency listed in Group A above, a patient can be considered to have AIDS if laboratory tests detect that he has been infected with HIV *and* if he has either a definitive diagnosis of any of the disorders listed in Group B above or a definitive or presumptive diagnosis of any of the disorders listed below.

With definitive diagnosis:
- HIV encephalopathy
- Kaposi's sarcoma
- HIV wasting syndrome.
- At least two recurrent bacterial infections over a 2-year period in a child under 13 years old. These include any combination of septicemia, pneumonia, meningitis, bone or joint infection, or abscess of an internal organ or body cavity caused by *Haemophilus, Streptococcus,* or other pyogenic bacteria. (Otitis media or superficial skin or mucosal abscesses aren't considered diagnostic.)
- Disseminated coccidioidomycosis at a site other than or in addition to the lungs or cervical or hilar lymph nodes
- Disseminated histoplasmosis at a site other than or in addition to the lungs or cervical or hilar lymph nodes
- Disseminated mycobacterial disease caused by other than *M. tuberculosis* occurring at a site other than or in addition to the lungs, skin, or cervical or hilar lymph nodes
- Extrapulmonary disease caused by *M. tuberculosis* involving at least one site, regardless of concurrent pulmonary involvement
- Recurrent *Salmonella* (nontyphoid) septicemia
- Isosporiasis accompanied by diarrhea that persists longer than 1 month
- Primary brain lymphoma
- Other non-Hodgkin's lymphoma of B-cell or unknown immunologic phenotype and either a small, uncleaved lymphoma of Burkitt or non-Burkitt type or an immunoblastic sarcoma (including immunoblastic lymphoma, large-cell lymphoma, diffuse histiocytic lymphoma, diffuse undifferentiated lymphoma, or high-grade lymphoma). *Note:* T-cell lymphomas aren't included here. Nor are lymphocytic, lymphoblastic, small-cleaved, or plasmacytoid lymphocytic lymphomas and histologically undescribed ones.

With presumptive diagnosis (employed only when definitive diagnosis is impossible):
- Candidiasis of the esophagus
- Cytomegalovirus retinitis with vision loss
- Disseminated mycobacterial disease involving at least one site other than or in addition to the lungs, skin, or cervical or hilar lymph nodes
- Kaposi's sarcoma
- Lymphoid interstitial pneumonia, pulmonary lymphoid hyperplasia, or both in a child under 13 years old
- *Pneumocystis carinii* pneumonia
- Toxoplasmosis of the brain affecting a child under 1 month old.

With laboratory evidence against HIV infection

If laboratory tests are negative for HIV infection, a diagnosis of AIDS for surveillance purposes is ruled out, unless:

- All causes of immunodeficiency listed in Group A above have been ruled out **and**
- The patient has had either *Pneumocystis carinii* pneumonia diagnosed definitively or any of the diseases listed in Group B above diagnosed definitively plus a T-helper cell count below $400/mm^3$.

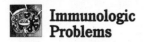

Acquired Immunodeficiency Syndrome

Continued

men. Between 1982 and 1987, the percentage of heterosexual women with AIDS increased 10%, while the percentage of heterosexual men with AIDS rose only 1%. The greatest risk factor for women is I.V. drug use. At least 50% of infected women probably use I.V. drugs; about 21% of infected women contracted the virus through sexual contact with an infected man.

Studying women with AIDS can provide a barometer for monitoring heterosexual transmission. It can also help predict future AIDS transmission to children, because women who are HIV-infected or who have AIDS are the main source of infection for infants. Nearly 80% of infected women are of childbearing age. And for every five women with AIDS, experts estimate that one child also has the disease.

CDC officials have been unable to determine the cause of about 4% of AIDS cases. In this group are patients whose risk information is incomplete because they've died or refused to be interviewed, patients still under investigation, patients who never returned for follow-up visits, men whose only reported high-risk behavior was having sex with a prostitute, and patients who don't seem to have any specific risk.

Transfusion recipients make up about 2% of AIDS patients. Hemophiliacs and people with other coagulation disorders make up an additional 1%. This relatively small group includes mostly people who received blood or blood products before 1985, when HIV blood screening began.

Assessment

When assessing a patient with possible HIV infection, be sure to evaluate his history, physical examination, and diagnostic tests. HIV infection can indirectly affect almost every body system, producing subtle and nonspecific changes in its early stages, possibly progressing to recurrent and fulminant complications in later stages. (See *How the CDC classifies HIV*, page 78.) Be sure to assess for opportunistic infections, malignancies, HIV encephalopathy, and HIV wasting syndrome. (See *HIV wasting syndrome*, page 78.)

Continued on page 78

Where AIDS hits hardest

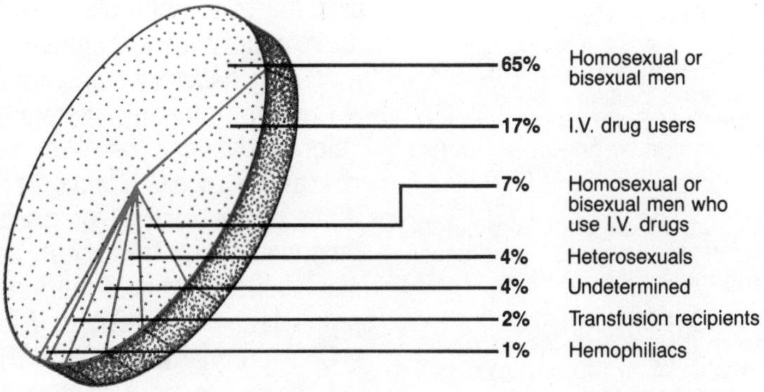

Acquired Immunodeficiency Syndrome

Continued

History. Start by taking a complete history, including the patient's chief complaint, present illness, past medical history, family history, and social history.

Chief complaint. The patient may report any number of nonspecific complaints, including fatigue, anorexia, weight loss, fever, night sweats, lethargy, dyspnea on exertion, depression, and diarrhea. Keep in mind, though, that some patients are asymptomatic until they abruptly develop a Kaposi's sarcoma lesion or symptoms of an opportunistic infection.

Present illness. Explore the patient's chief complaint and any other associated complaints. Find out when symptoms began, how long they've lasted, and how severe they seem. Ask about their location (if applicable) and about any factors that seem to precipitate or alleviate them.

Past medical history. Ask the patient if he's had similar symptoms in the past. If so, did he visit a doctor? What was the medical diagnosis and treatment? Find out if he's been hospitalized for any major acute or chronic illness; if so, record the course of the illness, its treatment, and any consequences.

Also ask the patient about medications. Is he using any prescription or over-the-counter drugs? Is he taking any experimental drugs? Record drug dosages and amounts, if the patient knows them, along with any adverse effects. Ask if he uses alcohol, recreational drugs, or "underground" remedies, because these can affect his response to treatment. Ask if he's allergic to any drugs, foods, or other agents. If so, ask him to describe his reaction.

Ask about characteristic symptoms, tailoring your questions to provide clues about the presence of secondary opportunistic infections, malignancies, and related conditions. Be sure to cover the following areas:

- Skin. Ask the patient if he's experienced poor skin turgor, dryness, or rash. Also ask if he's developed Kaposi's lesions, folliculitis, molluscum contagiosum, dermatitis, alopecia, local infections, or inflammation.
- Head and neck. Ask the patient if he's suffered hair loss, oral thrush, dental problems, cold sores or other oral lesions, or oral hairy leukoplakia. Ask about visual disturbances, retro-orbital pain, or changes in pupil size. Inquire about headaches, tinnitus, cranial nerve abnormalities, sinusitis, neck stiffness, and lymphadenopathy. (See *Lymphadenopathy syndrome*.)
- Cardiopulmonary system. Explore whether the patient has developed dyspnea or other respiratory problems, chest pain, dysrhythmias, pedal edema, orthopnea, cyanosis, or hemoptysis. Ask if he has a history of pneumonia. If so, ask about the kind of pneumonia, the treatment, and sequelae. If the patient's had PCP, ask about treatment and response and whether he's taking any prophylactic medications. Also ask when he last had a chest X-ray.
- GI system. Ask if the patient's had abdominal pain. If so, find out when the pain occurs, where it's located, how it feels, how severe it is, whether it radiates, and what seems to aggravate or alleviate it. Also ask about nausea and vomiting, anorexia, diarrhea

How the CDC classifies HIV

The Centers for Disease Control (CDC) classifies human immunodeficiency virus (HIV) infections in four groups.

Group I: Acute HIV infection
- Mononucleosis-like symptoms, possibly with aseptic meningitis
- HIV antibody in serum

Group II: Asymptomatic HIV infection
- No signs or symptoms of HIV infection
- HIV antibody in serum, but diagnostic tests may or may not reveal abnormal immune function

Group III: Persistent generalized lymphadenopathy
- Lymph nodes enlarged to 1 cm or more at two or more extrainguinal sites, persisting for more than 3 months
- No other illness to explain the lymphadenopathy

Group IV: Other HIV disease
- Signs and symptoms other than or in addition to lymphadenopathy:

Subgroup A. Constitutional disease—fever, weight loss, diarrhea
Subgroup B. Neurologic disease—dementia, myelopathy, peripheral neuropathy
Subgroup C. Secondary infectious diseases, such as *Pneumocystis carinii* pneumonia
Subgroup D. Secondary malignancies, such as Kaposi's sarcoma, that indicate acquired immunodeficiency syndrome (AIDS)
Subgroup E. Other conditions related to HIV infection or immunodeficiency; possible coexisting illness indicating immune defect.

HIV wasting syndrome

Sometimes called "slim disease," HIV wasting syndrome is characterized by severe, involuntary weight loss that exceeds 10% of the patient's baseline body weight. This weight loss must be accompanied by one of two other symptoms: chronic diarrhea (at least two loose stools a day for more than 30 days) or intermittent or persistent weakness and fever lasting more than 30 days.

Researchers are investigating whether the parasite *Microsporidia* might cause the severe diarrhea and weight loss associated with HIV wasting syndrome. Recent studies show that HIV may infect colon cells directly.

Acquired Immunodeficiency Syndrome

Lymphadenopathy syndrome

In this syndrome, also called persistent generalized lymphadenopathy, lymph glands in at least two extrainguinal sites swell to more than 1 cm and stay swollen for at least 3 months. If accompanied by fever, the condition is sometimes called lymphadenopathy-fever syndrome.

(when and how severe), esophageal pain or dysphagia, history of pancreatitis, hepatitis, and rectal lesions or bleeding. Determine if the patient has ever had a GI infection and, if so, when it occurred, the treatment he underwent, and any sequelae he suffered.

- Neurologic system. Find out if the patient has noticed any changes in his level of consciousness or motor, sensory, or gait disturbances. Ask if he's experienced peripheral neuropathies, symptoms of cranial nerve abnormalities, seizures, weakness in his extremities, paresis, or paralysis. Inquire about incontinence. Ask if he's fainted or noticed a lack of concentration or loss of memory. And ask if he has a history of meningitis or brain tumor.
- Hematologic system. Determine if the patient ever had anemia, leukopenia, or thrombocytopenia. Ask if he bruises easily, feels tired, or suffers frequent infections. Find out if his lymph nodes are swollen.
- Endocrine system. Ask if the patient has ever had symptoms of hypoglycemia, hyperglycemia, or hyponatremia.
- Genitourinary system. Ask if the patient ever had such sexually transmitted diseases as herpes simplex, syphilis, gonorrhea, hepatitis, or chlamydia. Find out if he's experienced dysuria, penile lesions (vaginal lesions in women), proctitis, Kaposi's sarcoma lesions, oliguria, or edema.

Family history. The patient's family history can point out environmental, genetic, or familial illnesses that might influence his current health problems or needs. Ask him about the general health of his blood relatives, spouse or companion, and sexual partners.

Social history. Environmental, psychological, and sociologic factors can profoundly affect a patient's mental and physical health, especially when AIDS is involved. If you suspect that a patient may be at high risk of HIV infection, try to get as complete a social history as possible. Ask about his occupation, cohabitants, the size of his family, and his home environment.

Tactfully obtain a sexual history. What risks has he incurred that might have exposed him to HIV infection? Is he currently sexually active? Are his partners predominantly male or female? What types of sexual activities does he engage in? Does he use condoms? Does he know and use safe sexual practices?

If the patient has AIDS, gently explore his fears and anxieties. Is he worried about losing his loved ones, his job, his insurance, or his independence? Has he felt increasingly depressed, irritable, or apathetic? Has he had insomnia, anorexia, or suicidal thoughts? Find out if he's ever been treated for depression.

Explore the patient's daily habits. How much and what does he usually eat? How much sleep does he need? Does he use tobacco or drink caffeinated beverages? Does he exercise and, if so, what kind of exercise does he do and how much?

Ask the patient about his support system. Does he have a companion or spouse? Is his family nearby? To whom does he usually turn when he's in trouble? Can he count on help from friends and family? Who's aware of his diagnosis, and whom does he plan to tell? If

Continued on page 80

Acquired Immunodeficiency Syndrome

Continued

he's homosexual, how many people know about it? How sensitive have people been so far? How much does he know about support groups in his community?

Assess the patient's financial status. Financial worries can add to his stress and exacerbate his condition. Consider asking your hospital's social worker to discuss the patient's financial concerns with him.

Throughout your nursing history, assess the patient's level of comprehension and cognition to help determine how much and what kind of health education he needs. Determine what he knows about HIV infection and its implications, and evaluate his response. You'll need to use this information when you're teaching the patient.

Physical examination. Begin by assessing the patient's vital signs. Be alert for fever and other signs of infection. Then thoroughly examine each body system.

Skin. Observe for poor skin turgor, lesions, rashes, cyanosis, and dermatitis. Check the skin around any venous access devices for inflammation.

Head and neck. Check for alopecia, temporal wasting, such oral lesions as oral hairy leukoplakia (about 80% of HIV-infected patients with oral hairy leukoplakia develop AIDS within 30 months), and thrush. Assess for Kaposi's sarcoma papules, dental abscesses, and gingivitis. Assess for cranial neuropathies, vision loss, neck rigidity, stomatitis, and anisocoria.

Neurologic system. Besides checking for cranial or peripheral neuropathies, assess for gait disturbances, extremity weakness, ataxia, hyperreflexia, paresis, paralysis, myoclonus, and signs of increased intracranial pressure. Also assess the patient's mental status and neurologic function. Check for signs of HIV encephalopathy (see *HIV encephalopathy*) and neurosyphilis.

Cardiopulmonary system. Assess for dysrhythmias, signs of cardiomyopathy or myocarditis, peripheral edema, and hypotension. Does auscultation reveal adventitious or decreased breath sounds? Does the patient have signs of tuberculosis?

GI system. Auscultate for abnormal bowel sounds. Check for abdominal pain, diarrhea, anal lesions or fistulas, bleeding, and signs of liver disease or hepatitis B infection.

Renal system. Assess for signs of renal disease.

Diagnostic tests. Patients with HIV infection must undergo multiple diagnostic tests. Described below are tests that may be used to establish an initial diagnosis of HIV infection, as well as diagnose associated opportunistic infections or malignancies.

HIV antibody tests. Two tests are commonly used to detect antibodies to HIV: the enzyme-linked immunosorbent assay (ELISA) and the Western blot assay. In the ELISA, the more common of the two, the patient's serum sample is incubated with live HIV. If HIV antibodies are present, they'll react with the test solution. An enzyme label

HIV encephalopathy

Also called HIV dementia, AIDS dementia, and subacute encephalitis, HIV encephalopathy is the most common neurologic effect of AIDS, occurring in 40% to 60% of affected patients. Its symptoms differ in severity, depending on the extent of CNS destruction.

Apparently, HIV preferentially attacks the brain's subcortical regions. This finding may mean that neurologic injury can be reversed. In fact, treatment with zidovudine has reversed the injury in some patients; in others, symptoms have reversed spontaneously.

In adults, diagnosis of HIV encephalopathy depends on the presence of cognitive or motor dysfunction (or both) severe enough to interfere with work or daily life. In infants and children, diagnosis may hinge on absence of normal developmental milestones. These findings unfold over weeks to months and exist with no concurrent illness besides HIV infection.

Early indications of HIV encephalopathy include:
- *Cognitive*—confusion, disorientation, impaired concentration and attention span, mental slowing, short-term memory loss
- *Behavioral*—apathy, delusions, hallucinations, impaired judgment, paranoia, restlessness and agitation, withdrawal
- *Motor*—dysarthria, gait ataxia, hyperreflexia, impaired handwriting, leg weakness, loss of coordination, psychomotor slowing, tremor, unsteady gait
- *Other*—anorexia, enuresis, hypersomnia, increased sensitivity to drugs and alcohol.

Late indications of HIV encephalopathy include circumlocution, confusion, disinhibition, distractibility, global dementia, organic psychosis, and coma. Ataxia, spasticity, hyperreflexia, myoclonus or seizures, paresis, or paralysis may occur. Psychomotor slowing may also be expressed as delayed verbal responses or near or absolute mutism. The patient may act unaware of his illness or stare vacuously; he may be incontinent.

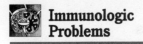

Acquired Immunodeficiency Syndrome

Diagnostic criteria for HIV

Because HIV infection poses unusual diagnostic problems, the Centers for Disease Control (CDC) has issued guidelines for achieving consistent diagnoses. Evidence that warrants a diagnosis of HIV infection includes any one of the following when the patient has a condition consistent with AIDS:

- In a patient over 15 months old—or in a child under 15 months old whose mother probably wasn't HIV-positive after birth—a serum specimen that's repeatedly reactive for HIV antibody in screening tests (enzyme-linked immunosorbent assay [ELISA], for example), followed by positive supplemental tests (Western blot or immunofluorescence assay, for example)
- In a child under 15 months old whose mother probably was HIV-positive after birth, a serum specimen that's repeatedly reactive for HIV antibody in screening and supplemental tests, plus increased serum immunoglobulin and at least one of the following abnormal test results: reduced lymphocyte count, reduced T-helper count, or decreased T-helper/T-suppressor ratio
- Positive test for HIV serum antigen
- Positive HIV culture, confirmed by both reverse transcriptase detection and a specific HIV-antigen test or in situ hybridization using a nucleic acid probe
- Positive results on any other highly specific HIV test.

Inconclusive evidence of HIV infection includes either one of the following:

- Repeatedly reactive screening tests for serum antibody to HIV, followed by negative or inconclusive supplemental tests without a positive HIV culture or serum antigen test
- In a child under 15 months old and born to a woman thought to be HIV-positive after birth, repeatedly reactive screening tests and possibly reactive supplemental tests, but without additional evidence of immunodeficiency and negative results on HIV culture or serum antigen test.

Evidence against HIV infection includes:

- Nonreactive screening tests and supplemental tests for serum antibody to HIV.

added to the serum and test solution detects the antigen-antibody reaction. ELISA can produce false-positive results, so any positive findings must be validated by a second ELISA. If this second test is also positive, a Western blot assay must be performed to confirm the results. This more definitive test can identify specific HIV antibodies.

Remember that positive test results indicate that a patient has been exposed to HIV and produced antibodies to it. Positive results don't mean that the patient has AIDS. (See *Diagnostic criteria for HIV.*) Conversely, negative results don't always mean the patient is free of HIV. For instance, if the patient was exposed to HIV just before the test, he may not have developed detectable antibody levels. He may carry HIV for several weeks to months before developing detectable levels. What's more, the ELISA test may not detect antibodies to HIV-2 infection.

Antigen test. This test, known as the HIVAGEN test, can detect antigens to HIV (HIV p24 core protein) as early as 2 weeks after infection. Research shows that patients who test positive for HIV antibodies and carry HIV antigen may be more apt to develop AIDS than patients who carry antibodies only. When HIV antigen appears along with HIV antibody, it indicates that the virus is actively replicating.

HIV culture. This procedure detects live HIV, but it can take up to 4 weeks. The test measures the amount of reverse transcriptase activity.

Several other tests may also be performed to detect malignancies and other complications. They include:

White blood cell count and differential. In AIDS, these tests show variable levels of immunosuppression that often correlate with the severity of clinical signs. Leukopenia is almost universal. Neutropenia often results from secondary infections or drug therapy, whereas lymphocytopenia occurs from destruction of lymphocytes by HIV. Thrombocytopenia also occurs frequently.

T-cell assay. Also known as an immune profile, this test measures the number of T cells. The extent of T-cell reduction usually parallels the disease stage. With HIV infection, the T-helper cell count usually declines while the T-suppressor cell count usually rises. Because of the destruction of T-helper cells following HIV infection, the normal ratio of T-helper to T-suppressor cells may reverse.

Cultures. Febrile HIV-infected patients may need frequent blood, urine, sputum, CSF, and other body fluid or tissue cultures. These tests help distinguish among the many secondary infections that can occur from immunosuppression.

Chest X-rays. These help detect pulmonary complications in febrile or dyspneic patients. If infiltrates appear on an X-ray, the patient may undergo bronchoscopy to detect PCP. Serial chest X-rays can help monitor response to therapy.

Continued on page 82

Acquired Immunodeficiency Syndrome

Continued

Pulmonary tests. Arterial blood gas studies and pulmonary function tests are routinely used to diagnose pulmonary complications and to monitor progress, especially in patients with PCP.

Tissue biopsy. This test can confirm a diagnosis of Kaposi's sarcoma.

Anergy profiles. Using a panel of recall antigens, these tests determine the integrity of the patient's cell-mediated immune response, which HIV infection severely affects. Most infected patients have these profiles repeatedly over the course of the disease.

Other tests. These include computed tomography (CT) scans, magnetic resonance imaging, gallium scans, and electroencephalography to diagnose and detect opportunistic infections, malignancies, and other complications or associated diseases.

Planning

Before determining your nursing care plan, develop the nursing diagnosis by identifying the patient's problem or potential problem, then relating it to its cause. Possible nursing diagnoses for a patient with AIDS include:

- infection, potential for; related to immunosuppression
- injury, potential for (trauma); related to weakness and confusion
- social isolation; related to abandonment by companions, friends, family
- knowledge deficit (HIV infection); related to inadequate patient teaching
- powerlessness; related to lack of control
- self-concept, disturbance in (self-esteem); related to diagnosis
- grieving, anticipatory; related to diagnosis outcome
- coping, ineffective individual; related to diagnosis
- nutrition, alteration in (less than body requirements); related to anorexia
- gas exchange, impaired; related to pulmonary infection.

The sample nursing care plan on page 83 shows expected outcomes, nursing interventions, and discharge planning for one of the nursing diagnoses listed above. However, you'll want to tailor each care plan to your patient's needs.

Intervention

Interventions for the AIDS patient include administering drugs to treat HIV infection and any related opportunistic infections and malignancies, providing supportive care, preventing transmission of HIV infection, providing psychosocial support, and providing patient and family teaching.

Administering drug therapy. Current therapy includes an anti-HIV drug to treat HIV infection and other agents to treat opportunistic infections and malignancies. Several drugs and an HIV vaccine are currently under investigation. (See *Investigational AIDS drugs*, page 84, and *HIV vaccine: On the horizon?*, page 85.)

Anti-HIV drug. Zidovudine (Retrovir), formerly known as azidothymidine (AZT), is the only drug that has received FDA approval for treating AIDS. The drug seems to directly inhibit HIV by interrupting the conversion of viral RNA into DNA before incorporation into the host

Diagnosing ARC

Diagnosis of AIDS-related complex (ARC) can be made if patients test positive for HIV antibody and show such nonspecific symptoms as chronic fatigue, progressive weight loss, persistent fevers, diarrhea, night sweats, anergy, generalized lymphadenopathy, and persistent minor infections. ARC patients may also have minor abnormalities in laboratory tests indicative of mild immunosuppression. They may go on to develop the full-blown effects of AIDS.

Acquired Immunodeficiency Syndrome

Sample nursing care plan: AIDS

Nursing diagnosis	**Expected outcomes**
Infection, potential for; related to immunosuppression	The patient will: • describe the signs and symptoms that can indicate an AIDS-related infection. • discuss methods of protecting himself from infection.
Nursing interventions	**Discharge planning**
• Assess for signs of infection, including fever, poor wound healing, and malaise. Notify the doctor of any such signs. • Teach the patient and his family about signs and symptoms of AIDS-related infection, including drenching night sweats, purple blotches or bumps on skin, white spots or patches in mouth, or persistent, unexplained fever, diarrhea, or weight loss. • Teach the patient and his family methods to prevent infection—for example, by careful handwashing; avoiding unpasteurized dairy products; cooking all raw vegetables, fruits, and meats before eating; avoiding direct contact with people who carry infectious disease; consulting the doctor about having a pet (because it may transmit opportunistic organisms); avoiding live vaccines; and maintaining good hygiene.	• Reinforce care plan with the patient and his family or caregivers. • Emphasize the importance of infection prevention. • Describe AIDS prevention measures, including safe sex practices. • Advise the patient about when to seek medical care. • Arrange for follow-up care, if needed.

cell's nucleus. However, it doesn't eliminate the virus, so treated patients can still carry the virus and may transmit it. Zidovudine crosses the blood-brain barrier and enters the CNS, so it might alter the course of infection.

Doctors generally prescribe zidovudine for patients with AIDS or severe manifestations of ARC who have a history of cytologically confirmed PCP or an absolute T-helper cell count under 200/mm^3. The recommended dose is 200 mg P.O. Because the drug has a short half-life, it must be given every 4 hours around the clock. Zidovudine's major adverse effect—bone marrow suppression—may lead to granulocytopenia and severe anemia, so patients may need frequent dose adjustments, transfusions, and meticulous monitoring of blood counts. Bacterial sepsis may occur as a result of secondary neutropenia. Caution patients taking zidovudine against using other drugs. Even acetaminophen can interfere with zidovudine metabolism.

Other agents. Besides undergoing therapy aimed at treating HIV infection itself, patients may also receive drugs to treat opportunistic infections (antimicrobial therapy) or malignancies (chemotherapy). Even with aggressive antimicrobial therapy, many opportunistic infections recur. Those involving the CNS or the eyes often require long-term therapy. Dosage, route, and treatment duration depend on the infection's location, the drug's adverse effects, the extent of hepatic or renal disease (common in AIDS), the tendency for the infection to recur and, possibly, the cost of therapy.

Continued on page 84

Acquired Immunodeficiency Syndrome

Investigational AIDS drugs

Dozens of drugs are being investigated for use in treating HIV infection and the opportunistic infections or malignancies associated with it. Most of these drugs are antivirals or immunomodulators. Phase III drugs are now in widespread clinical trials; Phase II drugs are being tested for effective doses; and Phase I drugs are being tested for safety. Here are some of the drugs from each phase.

Phase III	Phase II	Phase I	Others
• ABPP (bropirimine) • alfa-interferon (Wellferon) • ampligen (Poly IC12U) • eflornithine (DFMO, Ornidyl) • ganciclovir (Cytovene) • imreg-1 (Fleucocyte dialyzate) • imuthiol (Diethyldithiocarbamate) • thymopentin (TP5, Thymopoietin 32-36) • thymostimuline (TP-1)	• AL-721 • beta-interferon (Betaseron) • interleukin-2 (IL-2) • phosphonoformate (PFA, Foscarnet)	• acyclovir (Zovirax) • ansamycin (Rifabutine, LM-427) • anti-interferon immunoglobulin • CD4 (synthetic) • CL246,738 • colony stimulating factor (GM-CSF [granulocyte-monocyte colony stimulating factor] interleukin-3) • dideoxycytidine (DDC) • D-penicillamine (3-mercapto-D-valine) • gamma globulin (Hyperimmune) • gamma-interferon • immune globulin (IGIV) • methionine-enkephalin (MET-ENK) • muramyl-tripeptide (MTP-PE) • naltrexone (Trexan) • peptide T	These include AS-101, CS-85, erythropoietin, granulocyte colony stimulating factor, monocyte colony stimulating factor, and UA-100. Drugs whose clinical trials were suspended or have not been approved include HPA-23 (Antimonio-tungstate), isoprinosine (Inosine pranobex, inosiplex, methisoprinol), ribavirin (Virazole), and suramin.

Continued

The drugs listed below may be used to treat opportunistic infections. However, many of them are still experimental, so they may not be available at all hospitals. Antimicrobial therapy may include antifungal, antimycobacterial, antiviral, and antiprotozoal drugs.

Antifungal drugs. Commonly used in long-term therapy, antifungal drugs include oral preparations of nystatin and clotrimazole for oral candidiasis, and amphotericin B, 5-flucytosine, and ketoconazole for systemic or CNS fungal infections involving *Candida albicans, Cryptococcus neoformans, Histoplasma capsulatum,* or other pathogens.

Antimycobacterial drugs. Also used in long-term therapy, antimycobacterial drugs include such conventional antituberculars as isoniazid (Hyzid), rifampin (Rifadin), and ethambutol (Myambutol), and such experimental drugs as clofazamine and ansamycin. Experimental drugs are generally reserved for patients who don't respond to standard therapy.

Antiviral drugs. Included in this category are acyclovir, which is usually effective against herpes simplex infections, and the experimental drug ganciclovir (also called DHPG). Long-term therapy with ganciclovir may help prevent progressive pulmonary compromise or blindness when CMV infection results in pneumonitis or retinitis. Some doctors are now combining antiviral drugs and thymic tissue transplants. (See *Thymic tissue transplants: An attempt to restore immunity*.)

Antiprotozoal drugs. For treating toxoplasmosis, commonly prescribed antiprotozoal drugs include pyrimethamine, sulfadiazine,

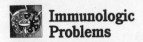

Acquired Immunodeficiency Syndrome

HIV vaccine: On the horizon?

Several HIV vaccines are now under development, two of which have been approved for testing by the Food and Drug Administration. Created through recombinant DNA technology, HIV vaccines usually consist of a form of the HIV envelope protein gp 160.

Investigators hope that HIV vaccines will stimulate production of HIV-neutralizing antibodies, and that the antibodies will then block viral proteins that usually bind to T-cell receptors. By preventing the virus from entering T cells, the vaccine could prevent HIV infection.

One problem with HIV vaccines so far has been an ethical one. Volunteers inoculated with the vaccine, who had previously tested HIV-negative, now test positive on ELISA and Western blot tests because they're producing anti–gp 160 antibodies. So, to prevent possible discrimination against them, test volunteers have been given documentation showing that they've been vaccinated and not infected with HIV.

Thymic tissue transplants: An attempt to restore immunity

Researchers are trying to restore AIDS patients' immune function by transplanting thymic tissue. So far, patients have shown a prompt, partial, selective, and transient repopulation of the circulating T-cell pool. What's more, the number of T8 cells, but not T4 cells, increased a few weeks after transplantation. These patients showed some clinical improvement.

Researchers doubt that thymic tissue transplants alone can revive the immune system. But they're hoping that transplants might be successful if coupled with antiviral drugs that block HIV replication.

or a combination of both. A reduced-folate supplement called leucovorin must be given concurrently because pyrimethamine interferes with folic acid metabolism.

For treating cryptosporidiosis, the experimental drug spiramycin may help ease the severe diarrhea associated with this infection.

For treating PCP, drugs of choice include trimethoprim-sulfamethoxazole (TMP-SMX) combination therapy and pentamidine isethionate. Many patients receiving TMP-SMX become sulfa-allergic, which often causes a rash after 6 to 10 days, requiring a switch to pentamidine. Besides possibly causing hypotension and dysrhythmias, pentamidine may also cause necrosis of pancreatic islet cells and increased serum insulin levels, possibly resulting in irreversible hypoglycemia or hyperglycemia. To reduce renal drug accumulation, researchers are administering pentamidine experimentally by aerosol inhalation. This route produces high drug accumulations in the lungs, and seems to be effective and nontoxic as both first-line and prophylactic therapy.

Another experimental drug—trimetrexate—proves effective for initial bouts of PCP and for treating patients intolerant or unresponsive to standard therapy. This drug inhibits dehydrofolate reductase, an enzyme produced by *Pneumocystis carinii*. Concurrent treatment with leucovorin is necessary to protect host tissues.

Other experimental drugs used for PCP include pyrimethamine, eflornithine (also called DFMO), dapsone, dapsone-trimethoprim, and BW 301. Studies are also underway to test TMP-SMX therapy as a way to prevent PCP.

Chemotherapeutic drugs. Chemotherapy is used to treat Kaposi's sarcoma and such other cancers as high-grade B-cell non-Hodgkin's lymphoma. Vincristine and vinblastine form the cornerstone of Kaposi's sarcoma treatment, although etoposide, doxorubicin, and alpha-interferon may also be used.

Providing supportive care. Besides drug therapy, patients with HIV infection or AIDS need considerable supportive care. Although HIV infection and AIDS progress differently from patient to patient, you'll usually need to intervene for the following problems:

- infection
- malnutrition
- mental status changes
- respiratory status changes
- elimination changes (especially diarrhea)
- skin breakdown
- pain
- chronic fatigue.

Infection. The type, location, and severity of opportunistic infections relate directly to the degree of a patient's immunosuppression. Starting antimicrobial drug therapy early can help prevent infection-related complications. But while antimicrobial drugs can help fend off opportunistic infections, they also can cause such complications as neutropenia, which may result in a gram-negative bacterial infection. Because antimicrobial drugs must be given in high doses

Continued on page 86

Acquired Immunodeficiency Syndrome

Continued

for a prolonged period, you'll need to assess their adverse effects frequently.

Antipyretics are commonly given to control high fevers, although acetaminophen should be avoided in patients on zidovudine. Fever with chills responds well to small doses of I.V. meperidine. Other measures include:

- providing adequate fluids to prevent dehydration
- ensuring adequate nutritional intake to meet increased metabolic demands
- preventing concurrent infections by maintaining sterile technique during invasive procedures; washing your hands carefully; protecting skin integrity by guarding against dryness and injury; promoting pulmonary hygiene; and inspecting catheter sites for localized edema, redness, and discharge.

Malnutrition. Meal planning may seem like a minor concern, considering the AIDS patient's overwhelming problems. But, in fact, malnutrition can contribute to the number and severity of opportunistic infections. Many AIDS patients have poor appetites and may suffer from weight loss of more than 10% and serum albumin levels under 2.5 g/dl. Malnutrition can develop in a patient with a symptomatic HIV infection for several reasons, including anorexia, dehydration, diarrhea, inadequate diet, infection, malabsorption, nausea and vomiting, and stomatitis. What's more, some drugs can cause nausea, alter food taste, or impair nutrient absorption.

To prevent malnutrition, emphasize the importance of increasing the patient's nutrient and caloric intake by eating more than normal. Encourage the patient to eat several small meals plus high-calorie, high-protein snacks throughout the day. To increase calories and nutrients, add dietary supplements such as Ensure, Isocal, and Polycose. Inquire about the patient's favorite foods, and ask your hospital's dietitian to provide them, if possible.

AIDS patients with severe diarrhea may have lactose intolerance, so arrange to have lactose-free foods for patients. Patients with oral candidiasis who have difficulty swallowing may need a soft diet or blender drinks. For patients suffering from nausea and diarrhea, provide medications as ordered. An antiemetic given 30 minutes before meals may be helpful. Topical anesthetic solutions, such as viscous lidocaine, as well as meticulous mouth care, can give relief to patients with stomatitis or painful oral lesions. Tell the patient to avoid tobacco, alcohol, and acidic or spicy foods; they can further irritate the oral mucosa, making nutrient intake even more difficult. If your patient's already malnourished, or if he simply can't consume enough calories, his doctor may start tube feeding or parenteral nutrition.

Mental status changes. HIV-infected patients may suffer such mental status changes as confusion, disorientation, mood or personality changes, poor judgment, or psychotic behavior. These changes may result from HIV invasion of the CNS, secondary brain infection or lymphoma, anoxia, fever, or drug toxicity.

Acquired Immunodeficiency Syndrome

You'll need to protect the confused or disoriented patient from injury. Safety measures include keeping side rails raised, restraining the patient if necessary, removing obstacles and sharp objects from his room, moving him to a room where he can be watched more closely, and keeping a small light on in his room at night. Also, remember to assess for visual changes, which could lead to blindness if caused by CMV. Posting "cue cards" around the room can remind a confused or forgetful patient to brush his teeth after meals and to perform other daily activities. Putting a calendar and a clock within easy view can also help orient the patient.

When talking to a confused patient, use short sentences and direct, simple language. Set limits, if necessary, and establish routines that he can follow easily and that lend structure to his life. If the patient has severe mental changes and is medically stable, his doctor may consider transferring him to a psychiatric care facility. You may need to discuss this with the health-care team and with his family; if so, do it as early as possible.

Respiratory status changes. AIDS patients can develop respiratory distress because of pneumonia, anemia, pleural effusion, postbronchoscopy pneumothorax, pain, activity intolerance, or Kaposi's sarcoma lesions of the tracheobronchial tree.

Oxygen therapy and appropriate antimicrobial drugs help treat respiratory complications. A humidifier can help loosen thick secretions. If fibrosis (a common sequela of PCP) is implicated in the dyspnea, teach the patient pursed-lip breathing. If he's taking bronchodilators, be sure he's using them correctly. Also teach relaxation techniques to ease the anxiety that accompanies dyspnea. As ordered, give morphine to reduce anxiety in a terminally ill dyspneic patient. Use of mechanical ventilation is controversial for an AIDS patient in respiratory failure.

Elimination changes. Diarrhea can develop from GI infection, malabsorption, metastasis to the GI tract by Kaposi's sarcoma, drug therapy, chemotherapy, or radiation therapy. Treatment should be directed at the underlying cause of the patient's diarrhea. Expect to withhold antidiarrheal medications until the cause of diarrhea becomes apparent. Treatment may involve antimicrobial drugs for GI infections, or radiation or chemotherapy for a malignancy that affects the GI tract.

Supportive care includes resting the bowel, monitoring fluids and electrolytes, giving I.V. fluids and nutrition, and encouraging bed rest. Patients may also benefit from a bland, low-fiber diet or a diet that doesn't include milk or milk products. Ambulatory incontinent patients can use incontinence pads to keep from becoming homebound. If diarrhea is excessive, assess the patient for fluid and electrolyte imbalance, and encourage him to drink fluids such as Pedialyte or Gatorade to prevent dehydration. In severe fluid and electrolyte imbalance, the doctor may order I.V. fluids.

Continued on page 88

Acquired Immunodeficiency Syndrome

Continued

Skin breakdown. In patients with AIDS, pressure sores or excoriation can be exacerbated by chronic genital *Candida* or anal herpetic lesions. Wash and air-dry the perineum and anal area regularly and apply prescribed ointments. If the patient is ambulatory, teach him to care for his lesions himself.

Pain. Pain can result from many factors, including abdominal cramping, anal lesions, anxiety, CNS involvement, dyspnea, edema, frequent invasive procedures, immobility, local infections, oral lesions, and fear. Expect to administer analgesic therapy and monitor to assess its efficacy. Many AIDS patients need pain medication administered on a schedule rather than as needed.

To help take your patient's mind off the pain, suggest such diversional and relaxing activities as guided imagery or listening to music with headphones. Massage, heat, and other topical treatments may also help, as may such adjunct therapies as psychotropic drugs, hypnosis, biofeedback, and yoga.

Chronic fatigue. Pulmonary insufficiency, infection, malnutrition, diarrhea, and depression can cause chronic fatigue. Suggest ways for patients to conserve their energy, including such measures as putting a tall stool in the kitchen so they can sit down while preparing meals, or putting a chair in the shower. Tell them to rest whenever they feel tired and to pace their activities.

Preventing HIV transmission. One of your most important tasks is teaching patients how to prevent transmission of HIV infection. This also includes taking precautions against contracting the infection yourself. The Surgeon General's Report, issued by the U.S. Public Health Service, offers sound guidelines for preventing transmission of HIV infection either through sexual contact or I.V. drug use. (See *Preventing AIDS transmission*.)

According to the report, heterosexual or homosexual couples who've maintained a mutually monogamous relationship for at least 5 years have little risk of acquiring HIV infection. But if any doubt exists regarding the fidelity of either partner, or about possible I.V. drug use by either partner, the couple must follow safe sexual practices. I.V. drug users must employ clean, fresh needles, syringes, and other equipment.

Health-care workers should follow CDC guidelines. Although occupational transmission has occurred, it's highly unlikely if you take the recommended precautions. Most important are strict blood and body fluid precautions, not just for patients with documented or suspected HIV infection, but for all patients. (See *Preventing HIV transmission in the health-care setting*, pages 90 and 91.)

Providing psychosocial support. Diagnosis of AIDS is a catastrophic event. It's associated with progressive deterioration and death, often within 2 years of diagnosis. But besides the disease itself, AIDS patients must face a type of fear and social stigma that few other dying patients encounter. With knowledge and sensitivity, you can help them through this difficult time. (See *Giving psychosocial support*, and *Explaining life-sustaining treatment issues*, page 92.)

Preventing AIDS transmission

To avoid AIDS transmission, provide these instructions to your patients:

- If you've been involved in any high-risk sexual activities or have injected I.V. drugs into your body without medical supervision, have a blood test to see if you've been infected with human immunodeficiency virus (HIV).
- If your blood test is positive, or if you take part in high-risk activities and decide not to be tested, inform your sexual partner. If you have vaginal or rectal sex, protect your partner by wearing a condom correctly from start to finish.
- If your sexual partner has an HIV-positive blood test, or if you suspect that your partner has been exposed to HIV, use a condom during sexual intercourse.
- If you or your sexual partner is at high risk, avoid oral contact with the penis, vagina, or rectum.
- Avoid all sexual activities that can cause cuts or tears in the linings of the penis, vagina, or rectum.
- Don't have sex with male or female prostitutes. Prostitutes, who are frequently I.V. drug users, can infect their clients through sexual intercourse; they can also infect other drug users by sharing I.V. drug equipment. Female prostitutes can also infect their unborn babies.

Acquired Immunodeficiency Syndrome

Giving psychosocial support

AIDS patients and their families need a great deal of support: emotional, social, and sometimes financial. Although every patient's needs differ, most can benefit from the following measures:

- Encourage your patient to express his feelings and concerns. Help him through the grieving process so he can learn to cope with his losses.
- Don't use the term "victim" around your patient because it implies defeat.
- Explain the reasons behind isolation precautions, so your patient won't feel shunned. Don't wear isolation garments when you're just talking or when you won't be in direct contact with body secretions.
- Stop to chat with the patient as much as possible. Encourage his family and friends to touch or hug him and to help with his care.
- Be tactful and sensitive when gathering personal data.
- Encourage the patient to join an AIDS support group, and be ready to help him make the initial contact.
- Encourage the patient to be as independent as possible so he can feel he has some control over his condition. Include him in all decision-making.
- If the patient seems severely depressed, discuss antidepressant therapy with the doctor.
- Arrange for flexible visiting hours so family and friends can spend as much time as possible with the patient.
- Advise the patient of his rights. Tell him he has the right to choose what types of treatment he wants, to have procedures explained to him, and to retain his privacy and the confidentiality of his medical information. He also has the right to refuse treatment, to refuse to participate in research, and to oppose discrimination shown against him because of his sexual preference or illness.
- If the patient needs financial assistance, have a social worker visit him soon after his hospitalization. Financial problems only add to the patient's feelings of powerlessness.

Patients cope with a diagnosis of AIDS in many ways, depending on their personalities and how they respond to other crises. Usually, any patient receiving a terminal diagnosis will go through three stages: crisis, transition, and acceptance.

Crisis. This phase, characterized by denial, begins when a person first learns he has a life-threatening disease. Denial can be a healthy buffer against reality until acute anxiety diffuses. Or it can be unhealthy, leading to complete disregard of medical advice. For example, an AIDS patient who denies his condition might continue to be sexually active without using precautions. Or he might continue sharing needles. Not only can these practices shorten the patient's own life, but they can endanger the lives of others as well.

Transition. Patients in this stage experience alternating feelings of anger, guilt, self-pity, and anxiety that overcome previous denial. Patients might obsessively review their past, trying to figure out how they contracted the infection or what they did to "deserve" AIDS. They might internalize negative societal attitudes about homosexuality and drug abuse and feel self-hatred. Homosexual men might even become homophobic.

Loss of privacy—actual or perceived—leads to feelings of anger. Patients fear losing their homes, jobs, health insurance, family and friends, and independence. Fear of losing independence increases as AIDS progresses and patients suffer chronic fevers, persistent weakness, dementia, and other debilitating problems. Patients know that eventually they may need help to accomplish even the most basic activities of daily living, perhaps requiring 24-hour care and supervision.

Feelings of isolation and loneliness can be as devastating as physical problems. A diagnosis of AIDS may force a homosexual man who hasn't already done so to "come out" to friends, co-workers, and family—and to possibly risk losing their love and support. Even if the patient's open about his homosexuality, he may feel that friends and loved ones will be fearful and angry when they learn of his illness, possibly abandoning him. Frequent hospitalizations only emphasize feelings of isolation. Hospital staff members have their own fears and prejudices, and they sometimes minimize contact with AIDS patients. Worse yet, patients often isolate themselves voluntarily, especially those with visible Kaposi's sarcoma lesions. Many avoid social activities and worry about transmitting the infection to others. They may also feel physically vulnerable, worrying about contagious diseases that could result from social contact. Isolation—either self-imposed or imposed by society—often leads to lingering depression; low self-esteem; insomnia; anorexia; anticipatory grief; and feelings of sadness, hopelessness, and worthlessness. Patients may withdraw completely from family and friends and begin to think of suicide, especially if they've had friends die of AIDS.

AIDS also may force patients to confront issues they're not emotionally prepared to face. Many AIDS patients are young, successful

Continued on page 91

Acquired Immunodeficiency Syndrome

Preventing HIV infection in the health-care setting

As the ranks of HIV-infected patients grow, the risk of exposure to infected blood grows too, especially for nurses and other caregivers. To reduce the infection risk, the Centers for Disease Control (CDC) urges that you treat all patients as if they were HIV-positive, even if you have no diagnostic information to support that premise. This approach is referred to as "universal blood and body-fluid precautions," or simply "universal precautions."

Following universal precautions eliminates the need for adhering to the blood and body-fluid (isolation) precautions previously recommended by the CDC for use with patients with known or suspected infections from blood-borne pathogens. Use isolation precautions as necessary for such associated conditions as infectious diarrhea or tuberculosis.

Universal precautions

- Use appropriate barrier precautions routinely to keep from exposing your skin or mucous membranes to patients' blood and some body fluids. Universal precautions do not apply to feces, nasal secretions, sputum, sweat, tears, urine, and vomitus unless they contain visible blood. Wear gloves when touching blood and indicated body fluids, mucous membranes, or broken skin; when handling items or surfaces soiled with blood or related body fluids; and when performing venipuncture and other vascular access procedures. Change gloves after contact with each patient. Also, be sure to wear a gown or apron and shield your face and eyes during procedures likely to generate droplets of blood or body fluids.
- Wash your hands and other skin surfaces immediately and thoroughly if they're contaminated by blood or body fluids. Wash your hands immediately after removing your gloves.
- Take precautions to prevent injuries caused by needles, scalpels, and other sharp instruments during procedures. Also take precautions when cleaning used instruments, disposing of used needles, and handling sharp instruments after procedures. To prevent needlestick injuries, don't recap needles, bend or break them by hand, or remove them from disposable syringes. After use, place disposable syringes and needles, scalpel blades, and other sharp items in puncture-resistant containers for disposal. Keep containers near the use area. Place large-bore, reusable needles in a puncture-resistant container for transport to the reprocessing area.
- Although saliva hasn't been implicated in HIV transmission (and may even reduce transmission, according to some researchers), it's wise to minimize the need for emergency mouth-to-mouth resuscitation by keeping mouthpieces, resuscitation bags, and other ventilation devices nearby.
- If you have exudative lesions or weeping dermatitis, don't give direct patient care or handle patient-care equipment until the condition resolves.

If you're pregnant, you're probably in no greater risk of contracting HIV infection than if you weren't pregnant. However, because you can transfer the virus to the fetus, you should be especially familiar with precautions and follow them closely.

Invasive procedure precautions

According to the CDC, an invasive procedure includes:
- surgical entry into tissues, cavities, or organs, or repair of major traumatic injuries, in a operating or delivery room, emergency department, or outpatient setting (including a dentist's office)
- cardiac catheterization or angiography
- vaginal or cesarean delivery or other obstetrical procedure where bleeding occurs
- manipulation, cutting, or removal of any oral or perioral tissues, including teeth, where bleeding occurs or the potential for bleeding exists.

For invasive procedures, follow the universal precautions as well as those listed below.
- Take barrier precautions with all patients. Always wear gloves and a surgical mask. For procedures that could cause splashing blood or body fluids, or flying bone chips, wear an apron or gown, and protective eyewear or a face shield.
- Wear gloves and a gown when handling the placenta or an infant during vaginal or cesarean delivery until blood and amniotic fluid have been removed from the infant's skin. Wear gloves while caring for the umbilical cord after delivery.
- If your glove tears or you get a needlestick or other injury, remove the old glove, and put on a new one as quickly as possible. Remove the needle or instrument from the sterile field.

Environmental precautions

Even though HIV doesn't seem to be transmitted environmentally, take the following precautions with all patients:
- Sterilize and disinfect all patient care equipment. HIV dies quickly after exposure to common chemical germicides, even at concentrations much lower than typically used. Besides commercial germicides, sodium hypochlorite (household bleach) is effective in concentrations of 1:100 to 1:10, depending on the amount of blood, mucus, or other material that needs to be removed from the surface being disinfected. Povidone-iodine is also effective.
- Clean the walls, floor, and other surfaces as usual; extraordinary measures aren't necessary.
- Clean and disinfect surfaces contaminated with blood and body fluids with chemical germicides approved for use as "hospital disinfectants." In patient care areas, remove visible material first, then decontaminate the area. Always wear gloves during cleaning and decontamination.
- When storing and processing soiled linen, handle it gently and as little as possible. Bag all soiled linen at the location where it was used; don't sort or rinse it in patient care areas. Put linen soiled with blood or body fluids in leakproof bags.

Dialysis precautions

HIV-infected patients with end-stage renal disease who are undergoing maintenance dialysis can be dialyzed using conventional infection-control precautions. Use universal precautions when dialyzing all patients.

Continued

Acquired Immunodeficiency Syndrome

Preventing HIV infection in the health-care setting—*continued*

Specimen collection and handling precautions

Consider blood and body fluids from all patients to be infectious. (In effect, this eliminates the need for warning labels on specimens; all specimens are considered infectious.)

Besides adhering to the universal precautions, follow these safeguards:
- When collecting the specimen, avoid contaminating the outside of the container or the laboratory form accompanying the specimen. Put all specimens in a sturdy container with a tight lid to prevent leakage during transport.
- Wear gloves when processing blood and body-fluid specimens. Wear a mask and protective eyewear if your mucous membranes might contact blood or body fluids. Change gloves and wash your hands after processing each specimen.
- Use a Class I or II biological safety cabinet for procedures likely to produce droplets, such as blending, sonicating, or vigorous mixing. A biological safety cabinet isn't necessary for routine procedures.
- Use a mechanical pipetting device for manipulating all liquids. Never pipette by mouth.
- Don't use needles and syringes unless absolutely necessary, and follow the recommendations for preventing accidental needlesticks.
- Cleanse work surfaces with an appropriate chemical germicide after spills of blood or body fluids and after work is finished.
- Decontaminate test materials before reprocessing them, or place them in bags and dispose of them following your hospital policy.
- Clean and decontaminate equipment contaminated with blood and body fluids before repairing it in the laboratory or transporting it to the manufacturer.
- Wash your hands and remove protective clothing before leaving the laboratory.

What to do if you're exposed

If you sustain parenteral exposure (such as a needlestick or cut), a mucous membrane exposure (such as a splash to the eye or mouth), or a cutaneous exposure involving large amounts of blood or prolonged contact (especially if the exposed skin is chapped, abraded, or has dermatitis), notify the patient of your exposure and request his consent for HIV testing. Consult hospital policy for testing patients who can't give consent, such as unconscious patients.

If the patient has AIDS, tests positive for HIV antibody, or refuses to be tested, you should seek counseling about the risk of infection and should undergo HIV testing as soon as possible. You should also report and seek medical attention for any acute, febrile illness occurring within 12 weeks of exposure. Such an illness can indicate recent HIV infection.

If initial test results are negative, have follow-up tests performed 6 weeks after exposure and at intervals thereafter, such as 12 weeks after exposure, and 6 months after exposure. Most people seroconvert during the first 6 to 12 weeks after exposure. During that period, assume that you may have the virus and take measures to prevent transmission.

If the patient is seronegative, you'll need no follow-up unless the patient is at high risk of HIV infection. In this case, you should be retested later (12 weeks after exposure, for example).

What to do if the patient's exposed

If the patient has parenteral or mucous membrane exposure to blood or body fluids from a health-care worker, inform him of the incident. Then follow the precautions outlined above.

Continued

people who were looking forward to the future. They simply aren't prepared for sickness and impending death.

Acceptance. Many patients eventually come to accept their diagnosis, its implications, and their death. While learning to accept the limitations AIDS imposes on them, they realize that they can still manage their lives. They become more reasonable and less emotional about their disease. They may turn to religion or other spiritual pursuits for comfort and hope. Patients might also find personal satisfaction in volunteering their time in AIDS support groups. At this point, they might take more responsibility for their own health, developing a fighting spirit and a renewed sense of hope for the future.

Providing patient and family teaching. Before teaching the patient and his family or caregivers, assess their motivation to learn, their anxiety level, and their ability to understand the information you'll present. This is especially important in a patient with HIV encephalopathy. Then evaluate how much the patient and his caregivers know about the following:
- HIV infection
- managment of the patient's signs, symptoms, and complications
- ways to reduce risk factors and prevent transmission
- community resources.

Continued on page 92

Acquired Immunodeficiency Syndrome

Continued

After explaining HIV infection, focus on how the infection affects your patient. Define immunosuppression and then explain opportunistic infections and malignancies and why the patient risks developing them. Your discussion should address the patient's current problems, those he's most likely to develop, and how they could be managed.

Explain how HIV infection can be transmitted. Try to determine and dispel any misconceptions held by the patient and his caregivers. Reassure them that HIV can't be transmitted by:
- hugging, social kissing, holding hands, or other nonsexual contact
- touching doorknobs, unsoiled linen or clothing, money, furniture, or other inanimate objects
- proximity to someone with AIDS at work, at school, in stores, in restaurants, in elevators, or in other public places
- toilet seats, bathtubs, showers, or swimming pools
- dishes, silverware, or food handled by an infected person
- animals or insects (although animals do carry other infections transmissible to immunosuppressed people).

Emphasize that HIV dies quickly outside the body because it needs living tissue to survive. Explain that the virus is easily killed by soap, cleansers, hot water, and such disinfectants as household bleach.

Explain how HIV is transmitted: through intimate sexual contact, direct inoculation into the bloodstream (such as during I.V. drug use or accidental needlestick), or perinatally from an infected mother. If a caregiver becomes exposed to the patient's blood, he should wash with soap and water immediately. To minimize the risk of transmission, advise the patient not to:
- donate blood, plasma, body organs (including eyes and corneas), tissues, or semen
- share needles, syringes, or such personal items as toothbrushes or razors that might carry blood or body fluids
- be shaved by a barber
- get tattooed
- become pregnant
- use recreational drugs, because they may have immunosuppressive effects
- receive care from a doctor, nurse, or dentist without first indicating he has AIDS or is HIV-positive
- have unprotected sexual intercourse.

Take time to discuss safe sexual practices with your patient. Tell him that these include hugging, petting, massaging, mutual masturbation, social kissing, using sex toys, and having protected sexual intercourse. (See *Tips for condom use.*)

Advise your patient to avoid the following unsafe sexual practices:
- receptive or insertive anal intercourse without a condom
- vaginal intercourse without a condom
- fellatio without a condom
- cunnilingus
- insertion of a fist or foreign object into the rectum
- oral-anal stimulation.

Explaining life-sustaining treatment issues

AIDS patients typically suffer a number of medical crises before succumbing to the disease. For this reason, you'll need to gently discuss resuscitation issues with your patient early in his hospitalization—before a medical crisis forces the issue, and while the patient's still able to communicate his wishes.

Explain the meaning of resuscitation and advanced life support. Tell the patient that it's his right to decide what life-sustaining measures he wants. Reassure him that being allowed to "die naturally" doesn't mean the end of pain control, comfort measures, or emotional support.

Also tell the patient how to document his wishes about life-sustaining treatment in a living will, if your state recognizes them. Or he can designate a proxy (preferably a family member or close friend) to make decisions for him if he becomes incompetent. Called durable power of attorney, all states recognize this option.

In any case, encourage him to put his wishes in writing and have them witnessed or notarized. Otherwise, the courts can appoint a legal guardian for him if he becomes incompetent. If your patient's homosexual, he should also know that the courts usually don't recognize homosexual relationships. So if he wants his companion to act on his behalf, he must have the companion appointed as his legal guardian.

Acquired Immunodeficiency Syndrome

Tips for condom use

Short of abstinence, condoms provide the best protection against sexual transmission of HIV. However, they give little or no protection if used incorrectly. Provide your patients with these tips for using condoms:
- Use a condom every time you have oral, anal, or vaginal sex.
- Use latex condoms instead of "natural" ones; they give better protection.
- Open wrappers carefully; a jagged fingernail can tear the condom.
- Lubricate inside the tip of the condom with plain water or a water-based lubricant, such as K-Y jelly, to increase sensation without allowing slippage. You can also use spermicidal jelly or foam containing nonoxynol-9, which kills HIV. Don't use oil-based products, such as mineral oil, cold cream, or petroleum jelly, because they can weaken the latex.
- To apply a condom, retract the foreskin, if necessary, and unroll the condom over the entire erect penis. Press out the end of the condom tip to remove air bubbles. When using plain-end condoms, keep a half-inch free at the end to collect sperm.
- Add extra water-based lubricant to the outside of the condom before entry. Inadequate lubrication can cause condoms to tear or pull off. If the condom begins to slip during intercourse, hold the base with your fingers.
- After ejaculation, hold the condom's base and withdraw before losing the erection. If the erection subsides, the condom may slip off, allowing semen to escape.
- Never reuse a condom.
- Store unused condoms in a cool, dry place because heat can damage the latex.

Finally, teach the patient and his caregivers how to prevent opportunistic infections and other complications. For example, the patient should:
- avoid unpasteurized milk or milk products
- avoid "organic" foods
- fully cook all meats, fruits, and vegetables before eating
- avoid direct contact with people who have contagious illnesses
- ask a doctor if it's safe to have a pet, because some animals carry the intestinal parasites *Cryptosporidium* and *Toxoplasma*, which cause severe infection in AIDS patients
- avoid touching animal feces, urine, emesis, litter boxes, aquariums, or bird cages, because they may harbor opportunistic organisms
- avoid live-virus vaccines, which can be fatal to immunosuppressed people
- exercise regularly
- control stress
- stop smoking to minimize respiratory problems
- practice safe sex to avoid transmitting the virus and contracting secondary infections.

Evaluation

Base your evaluation on the expected outcomes listed on the nursing care plan. To determine if the patient has improved, ask yourself the following questions:
- Does the patient show signs of infection?
- Can he describe the signs and symptoms of an AIDS-related infection?
- Does he know how to protect himself from further infection?
- Does he know when to seek medical attention?
- Does he know how to prevent transmission of the virus to others?
- Does he understand how to practice safe sex?

The answers to these questions will help you evaluate your patient's status and the effectiveness of his care. Keep in mind that these questions stem from the sample nursing care plan on page 83. Your questions may differ.

Pediatric AIDS

More than three-fourths of the children who've contracted AIDS so far have received it perinatally from their mothers; the remainder received infusions of HIV-contaminated blood. So far, no children have contracted the disease as a result of sexual abuse.

Although the exact transmission route isn't always clear, the virus travels to a fetus or infant in one of three ways:
- across the placenta before birth
- from the mother's body fluids during birth
- from infected breast milk after birth.

So far, most mothers who've infected their infants have been I.V. drug users but, as more women contract AIDS through heterosexual intercourse, this route of transmission promises to grow more common.

Continued on page 94

Acquired Immunodeficiency Syndrome

How pediatric AIDS compares to adult AIDS

Children with AIDS may present a strikingly different clinical picture than adults with AIDS. For instance, pediatric patients rarely develop Kaposi's sarcoma, B-cell lymphoma, or acute mononucleosis-like symptoms. They also don't usually develop hepatitis B or peripheral lymphopenia.

Pediatric AIDS patients do, however, experience problems that are uncommon or milder in affected adults. These include hypergammaglobulinemia, lymphoid interstitial pneumonitis, serious bacterial infection, and progressive neurologic disease caused by central nervous system infection. Pediatric patients may also have dysmorphic facial features. What's more, they may exhibit a normal ratio of T-helper to T-suppressor cells, although there will be fewer T-helper cells than normal.

Pediatric AIDS—*continued*

Children who've contracted HIV infections from blood transfusions either had medical problems requiring transfusions during the neonatal period or had hemophilia or another coagulation disorder. Now that blood undergoes rigorous testing before use, virtually all children who contract AIDS in the future will acquire it perinatally from their mothers. Some experts predict that as many as 65% of children born to HIV-seropositive mothers will become infected with the virus perinatally.

Many pediatric patients succumb to bacterial infection (particularly gram-negative sepsis) or other opportunistic infection. Infants showing symptoms of HIV infection before their first birthday and those who develop PCP have poor long-term prognoses. However, a small number of children seem to fare better than adults. Those with a different type of pneumonia—lymphoid interstitial pneumonitis (LIP)—have lived as long as 6 years after diagnosis. (See *How pediatric AIDS compares to adult AIDS.*)

Assessment

The history, physical examination, and diagnostic tests are basically the same for a child as they are for an adult.

History. Ask the child's parents about his present illness and medical history, as well as about possible risk factors. For example, ask if anyone in the family had a blood transfusion before 1985, if either parent uses I.V. drugs, if the father is bisexual, or if the mother is a prostitute. Keep in mind that the parents could be carrying HIV without realizing it; many times, the child is the first family member diagnosed with AIDS.

Physical examination. Failure to thrive is a primary sign of AIDS in infants. This poor growth can result from malabsorption syndrome or infections. Other common problems include lymphadenopathy, hepatosplenomegaly, and persistent oral thrush. Many patients also have developmental delays or loss of developmental milestones.

Evaluate the patient for signs of bacterial infection, which can become systemic and impair CNS function. Neuropathy can also stem from HIV infection of neural tissue. Bacterial infections that can produce otitis media and progress to septicemia include those caused by *Salmonella, Mycobacterium avium-intracellulare*, and other gram-negative bacteria.

Be sure to assess for signs of PCP, LIP, and Candida esophagitis. LIP, more common in children than adults, causes lymphocytes lining the lungs' alveoli to overgrow, resulting in a persistent, dry, hacking cough. Children with LIP may survive longer than those with PCP because their immune systems function to some extent.

Almost all children with AIDS have CNS involvement. Assess for chronic encephalopathy, which can result from viral or bacterial infections (from *Toxoplasma, Cryptococcus, Mycobacterium avium-intracellulare*, or CMV) or as a direct result of primary HIV infection. Children with AIDS usually have chronic, severe diarrhea. Possible causative organisms include *Cryptosporidium, Giardia lamblia, Sal-*

Acquired Immunodeficiency Syndrome

Guidelines for pediatric HIV testing

These guidelines are suggested by various San Francisco medical agencies involved in AIDS prevention and research.

- Infants born to HIV-infected mothers should be tested for HIV antibody at 1 year, after passively acquired maternal antibodies have disappeared. Infants showing symptoms before reaching 1 year should be tested immediately and, if possible, have a viral culture to confirm HIV infection.
- Infants born to high-risk mothers whose prenatal antibody status isn't known should be tested before reaching 2 months old and again at 1 year. If they develop symptoms before this time, they should be tested immediately.
- Foster children at least three years old and born after 1978, especially to high-risk mothers, should be tested if they show marked neurodevelopmental delay, lack of control over body secretions, such aggressive behavior as biting, or oozing lesions.
- Children available for adoption and born after 1978, especially those at high risk of HIV infection, should be tested. Results should be made available to adoptive parents before final placement.

monella, Candida, Mycobacterium avium-intracellulare, Microsporidia, Isospora belli, CMV, and HIV.

Tumors don't commonly occur in pediatric AIDS patients, although Kaposi's sarcoma and brain cell lymphomas have been reported. However, some pediatric patients develop cardiomyopathy leading to congestive heart failure.

Some researchers believe that infants infected in utero also show dysmorphic features such as microcephaly; hypertelorism; a prominent, boxlike forehead; a flattened nasal bridge; mildly oblique eyes; and others. This theory is controversial. (See *Dysmorphic features in pediatric AIDS*, page 96.)

Diagnostic tests. Diagnosing AIDS is more difficult in infants than in older patients. Because the majority of infants contracted AIDS perinatally, they'll carry antibodies to HIV, acquired passively before birth, for up to 15 months.

Other diagnostic tests performed on infants and children are the same as those performed on adults. Test results have shown hypergammaglobulinemia (or, in some cases, extreme hypogammaglobulinemia), depressed T-helper cells, leukopenia, thrombocytopenia, reversed lymphocyte subset ratio, depressed lymphocyte responses to mitogens, increased circulating immune complexes, decreased specific antibody responses, and elevated serum transaminase levels. Children with AIDS also typically test positive for CMV, Epstein-Barr virus, and hepatitis B. CT scans of children with chronic neurologic changes show basal ganglia calcifications and cortical tissue atrophy.

Intervention

Interventions are basically the same as those for the adult AIDS patient. They include drug therapy, supportive care, transmission prevention, psychosocial support, and patient and family teaching. An acutely ill child should receive immediate symptomatic care. If he survives the acute illness, long-term care and follow-up become priorities. Overall goals include physical care for the child and prevention of HIV transmission.

Drug therapy. Experimental drugs are being used to treat HIV infection in infants and children as well as in adults. However, viral CNS infections leading to neuropathy are common in HIV-infected children. Therefore, only drugs capable of crossing the blood-brain barrier to fight viral CNS infections should be considered for experimental use in children.

One drug that's been given intravenously in infants and children is hyperimmune serum, although it hasn't been proven to control HIV infection. This drug has also been administered early in pregnancy to women infected with HIV, possibly to prevent transplacental transmission to the fetus. Two combination treatments are being tested. The first combines two antiviral agents: zidovudine and ribavirin. Some antagonism exists between these drugs, how-

Continued on page 96

Acquired Immunodeficiency Syndrome

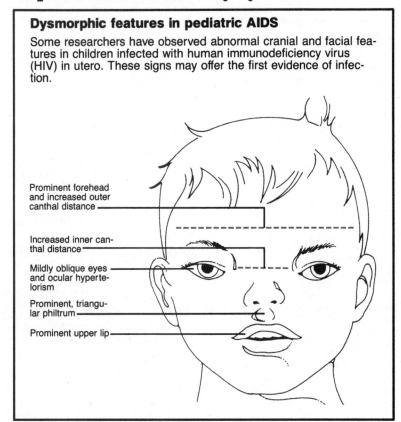

Dysmorphic features in pediatric AIDS

Some researchers have observed abnormal cranial and facial features in children infected with human immunodeficiency virus (HIV) in utero. These signs may offer the first evidence of infection.

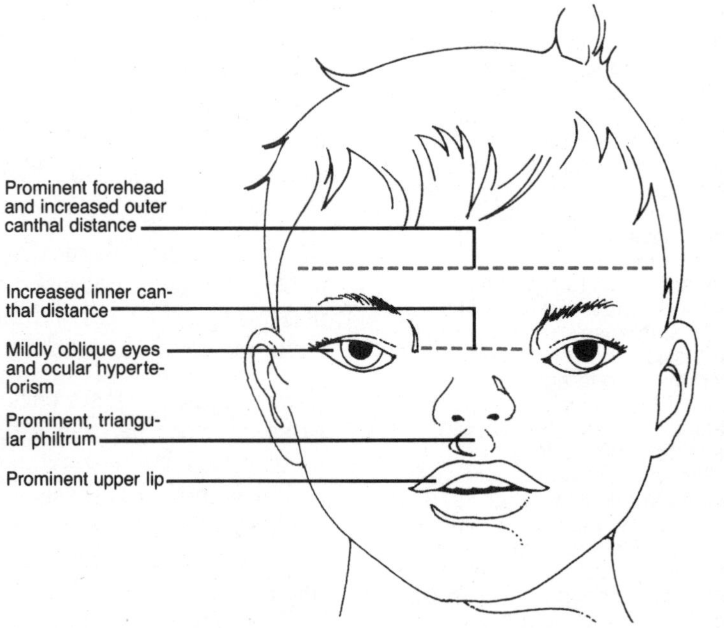

Special precautions for pediatric AIDS patients

Pediatric AIDS patients need special care, including:

Vaccines
Give only killed vaccines. Notify the doctor if an HIV-positive child will be in close contact with newly vaccinated children.
- Avoid giving HIV-infected children tubercular vaccines containing bacille Calmette-Guérin, or vaccines for measles, mumps, or rubella. You can administer such inactivated vaccines as *Haemophilus influenzae* Type B and pertussis as well as diphtheria and tetanus toxoids on schedule.
- Give an inactivated polio vaccine rather than the activated oral form. Administer polio vaccines along with pertussis vaccine and diphtheria and tetanus toxoids at 2, 4, 6, and 18 months, and 4 to 6 years of age.
- Be sure that older high-risk children undergo testing for HIV exposure before receiving live-virus vaccines. If the parent or guardian won't allow testing, don't inoculate the child.

Fevers
Children with AIDS can run fevers of 101° to 105° F. (38.3° to 40.6° C.) for weeks. If tests don't reveal a bacterial infection, the cause is assumed to be HIV.
- Keep the child warm and comfortable, change the bed linens often, and use extra blankets.
- Give sponge baths and fluids to control fever.
- Clean the thermometer after each use and don't use it for any other family members.
- If the child has chronic diarrhea, take his temperature under his arm rather than rectally.

Nutrition
Give a high-calorie, high-protein diet that supplies 100% to 150% of the recommended daily allowance for the child's weight. Tell parents to increase caloric intake and food appeal.

Blood products
Irradiate blood or blood products to be given to children with HIV infection, ARC, or AIDS to prevent graft-versus-host disease.

Umbilical stumps
Clean umbilical stumps of seropositive infants daily until they fall out or are removed.

Circumcision
HIV-infected babies shouldn't be circumcised because it can lead to infection.

Pediatric AIDS—*continued*

ever, so studies are proceeding cautiously. The second treatment combines an antiviral agent with an immunoenhancing one, to strengthen immune function without activating HIV. Other experimental treatments include using thymic hormone-fraction V to temporarily improve T-cell function, and using gamma globulin infusions every 2 to 4 weeks to help prevent recurring infections.

Opportunistic infections in infants and children usually require the same drugs used for adults; however, recurrent bacterial infections are a major problem in children with AIDS. Optimal antibiotic therapies haven't been established yet.

Supportive care. Like that for adults, supportive care for infants and children with AIDS consists of:
- avoiding infection
- preventing or treating malnutrition
- maintaining skin integrity
- dealing with pain and chronic fatigue
- managing mental status, respiratory, and elimination changes (especially diarrhea).

Preventing HIV transmission. In children as well as adults, transmission prevention focuses on avoiding infected blood and body fluids during patient care. Parents, caregivers, and all others must follow the CDC guidelines outlined earlier in the chapter.

Keep in mind that the immunosuppressed child is more at risk of catching a secondary infection than a healthy child is of contracting

Acquired Immunodeficiency Syndrome

HIV. In fact, because the virus spreads only through sexual contact or contaminated blood or body fluids, the chance of another child acquiring the infection is remote. Naturally, the amount of interaction between the pediatric AIDS patient and other children depends on the child's age, developmental stage, and level of understanding.

Psychosocial and educational interventions. Families of HIV-infected children need a great deal of support and education. Your teaching should cover three main points: how to care for the child, how to prevent transmitting the disease to other family members, and how to control opportunistic infections.

Teach the parents how to administer medications, what signs and symptoms of infection to watch for, and how to control fever. (See *Special precautions for pediatric AIDS patients*.) Explain that caregivers should wear disposable gloves when changing diapers, cleaning wounds, or risking contact with blood or body fluids.

Once a child is known to be HIV-positive, the family needs close follow-up and counseling. Because these families often belong to lower socioeconomic groups, you'll need to assess the family support system. Urge other family members to be screened for the HIV antibody. If one or both parents are drug addicts, provide information on drug rehabilitation. If one or both are HIV-positive, counsel them on safe sexual practices, and advise the mother about the danger of having another HIV-positive baby. Also tell the parents about needed services, such as a hospice, that may be available in their community. Maintaining patient confidentiality is essential.

Primary and Secondary Immunodeficiency Disorders: Preventing Infection

Joyce P. Griffin, who wrote this chapter, is an assistant professor of nursing at the University of Hawaii. Dr. Griffin received her BSN from the Herbert Lehman College of the City University of New York, her MSN from the Hunter College of the City University of New York, and her PhD from New York University.

In this chapter, we'll discuss disorders that develop when elements of the immune system function inadequately or are altogether unresponsive. Whether congenital, acquired, or iatrogenic, immunodeficiency disorders heighten susceptibility to infection, sometimes from organisms that aren't usually pathogenic.

Much of your nursing care for immunodeficient patients will consist of recognizing, treating, and preventing life-threatening infections as well as providing emotional support. This chapter begins with a general discussion of immunodeficiency and includes a review of the signs, symptoms, and interventions associated with selected immunodeficiency disorders.

Defining immunodeficiency

When a patient develops an immunodeficiency disorder, it indicates an impairment in one or more of the major mechanisms of host defense:

- antibody-mediated (B-cell) immunity
- cell-mediated (T-cell) immunity
- phagocytosis
- complement.

Immunodeficiency disorders can be grouped into two categories: primary and secondary. *Primary immunodeficiency disorders* stem from intrinsic defects in the development of immunocompetent cells. These disorders may be congenital or acquired. *Secondary immunodeficiency disorders* arise from such external factors as disease (malignancy or malnutrition, for example), from certain therapies (radiation or chemotherapy, for example), or both.

Primary immunodeficiency disorders

Both congenital and acquired primary immunodeficiency disorders have their origin in defects at various points along the differentiation pathways of immunocompetent cells or in defects in components of the immune system. These defects may result from an embryologic abnormality caused by enzymatic defect or from an unknown cause. (See *How primary immunodeficiency disorders develop*.) Defects may involve:

- primary development of T cells or B cells
- the antigen-dependent phase of B-cell or T-cell differentiation
- secondary B-cell differentiation
- phagocytes or complement.

Severe forms of primary immunodeficiency usually appear early in life and frequently end in childhood death. However, patients may acquire an immunodeficiency disorder at any age, and a substantial number survive to middle age or beyond. Scientists classify immunodeficiency disorders according to mode of inheritance and whether the defect involves T cells, B cells, or both.

Assessment

Primary immunodeficiency disorders leave patients highly susceptible to infection and sometimes to autoimmune disease and lymphoreticular malignancies. When obtaining the patient's history or performing a physical examination, be alert for signs of infection. (See *Signs of immunodeficiency*.) If infection is present, accurately

Continued on page 100

Signs of immunodeficiency

Strong indicators of immunodeficiency include:

- chronic or unusual infections
- poor response to treatment
- recurrent infection, especially with incomplete recovery between bouts.

Probable indicators of immunodeficiency include:

- delayed infant development
- hepatosplenomegaly
- persistent diarrhea
- rash, especially eczema or candidiasis
- recurrent abscesses or osteomyelitis
- signs of autoimmunity.

Indicators of specific immunodeficiency disorders include:

- ataxia
- cartilage-hair hypoplasia
- eczema
- idiopathic endocrinopathy
- partial albinism
- short-limbed dwarfism
- telangiectasia
- tetany
- thrombocytopenia.

Primary and Secondary Immunodeficiency

How primary immunodeficiency disorders develop

Antibody- and cell-mediated immunodeficiencies can result from several developmental defects that interrupt cell maturation.

Combined immunodeficiencies occur when congenital or acquired factors impede stem cell differentiation into B cells and T cells.

Deficiencies can also occur when T cells are blocked from migrating to or from the thymus, or when B cells are blocked from migrating to the bursal equivalent tissue.

Blocked antibody synthesis may also cause an immunodeficiency disorder.

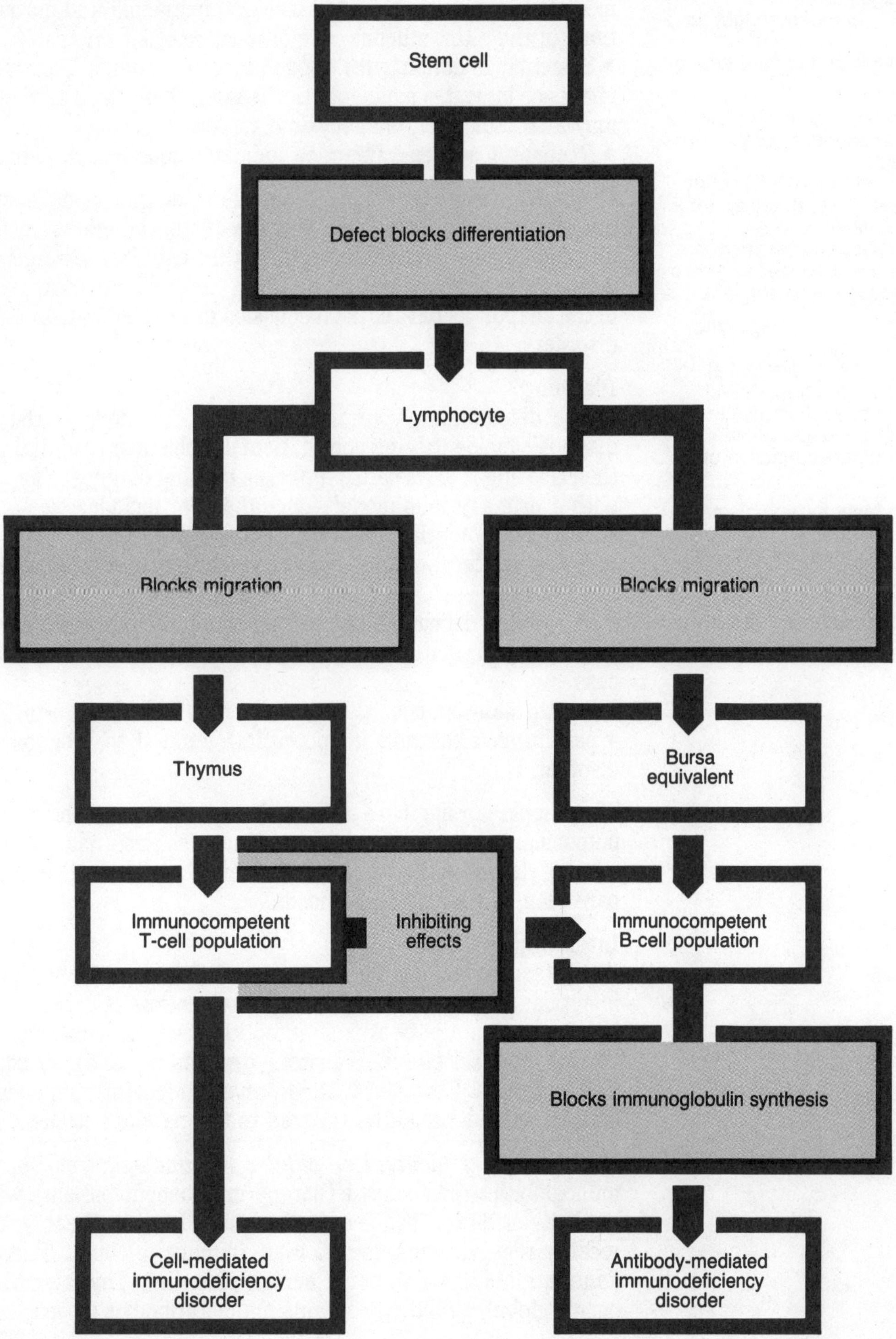

Primary and Secondary Immunodeficiency

Primary immunodeficiency disorders—*continued*

tracking its course may help to identify the specific immunodeficiency disorder and evaluate its severity.
- Recurrent bacterial sinopulmonary infections, such as otitis media and pneumonia, indicate defective antibody-mediated immunity.
- Fungal, protozoal, and viral infections may indicate defective cell-mediated immunity. Findings include pneumonia and chronic infections of the skin, mucous membranes, or other organs.
- Systemic infection with pyogenic or uncommon bacteria of low virulence indicates a phagocytic disorder. Superficial skin infections may also indicate a phagocytic disorder.
- Recurrent pyogenic infection indicates complement deficiencies.

Diagnostic tests. Screening tests allow diagnosis of most immunodeficiency disorders. More complex tests, though not available in all laboratories, can help diagnose the rest. (See *Screening for immunodeficiency disorders*.) Information on specific tests appears later in the chapter as part of the discussion of selected immunodeficiency disorders.

Planning

Before determining your nursing care plan, develop the nursing diagnosis by identifying your patient's problem or potential problem, then relating it to its cause. Possible nursing diagnoses for a patient with a primary immunodeficiency disorder include:
- infection, potential; related to immunosuppression
- coping, ineffective family (compromised); related to altered growth and development
- knowledge deficit; related to inadequate health teaching
- self-concept, disturbance in (body image); related to disease process
- health maintenance, alteration in; related to long-term therapy
- parenting, alteration in (potential); related to prognosis of the disorder.

The sample nursing care plan on the opposite page shows expected outcomes, nursing interventions, and discharge planning for one nursing diagnosis listed above. However, you'll want to tailor each care plan to your patient's needs.

Intervention

Key interventions include prompt, aggressive antibiotic therapy for infections and, at times, protective or reverse isolation. Such isolation protects a patient from infectious organisms carried by hospital staff, other patients, visitors, droplets in the air, or equipment and materials. However, it can't prevent infection from endogenous organisms and should be tailored to the patient's needs.

Replacement of humoral or cellular immunologic components. Immunoglobulin replacement therapy may benefit patients who have antibody-mediated deficiency disorders. In this therapy, patients receive regular administration of immune globulin (also called gamma globulin or immune serum globulin). This sterile, nonpyogenic globulin solution contains many antibodies normally present

Screening for immunodeficiency disorders

Screening tests for antibody-mediated (B-cell) immunodeficiencies include:
- IgG, IgM, and IgA levels
- isohemagglutinin titer (anti-A and anti-B), to measure IgM function
- Schick test, to measure IgG response.

Screening tests for cell-mediated (T-cell) immunodeficiency disorders include:
- white blood cell (WBC) count with differential, to measure total lymphocyte level
- delayed hypersensitivity skin tests, to measure T-cell and macrophage response to antigens.

Screening tests for phagocytic disorders include:
- WBC count with differential, to measure total neutrophil level
- nitroblue tetrazolium dye test and chemiluminescence, to measure the metabolic function of neutrophils.

Screening tests for complement disorders include:
- C3 level, to measure most important complement component
- hemolytic complement level, to quantitate complement activity.

Primary and Secondary Immunodeficiency

Sample nursing care plan: Primary immunodeficiency disorder

Nursing diagnosis	Expected outcomes
Infection, potential for; related to immunosuppression	The patient will: • show no signs of infection. • learn methods to prevent infection. • recognize the signs of infection. • understand the importance of preventing infection.
Nursing interventions	**Discharge planning**
• Reduce the patient's risk of infection by: —washing your hands thoroughly before and after care —wearing gloves during care —maintaining reverse isolation and monitoring visitors. • Obtain and record patient's temperature at least every 4 hours. Report fever immediately. • Monitor WBC count and report elevations or depressions. • Obtain cultures of urine, respiratory secretions, wound drainage, and blood, as indicated. • Urge patient to wash his hands before and after meals and after using the bathroom, bedpan, or urinal. Help him keep perianal area clean after elimination. • Offer oral hygiene every 4 hours to prevent bacterial growth and avoid descending infection. • Use strict aseptic technique when suctioning the lower airway, inserting urinary or I.V. catheters, and providing wound care. • Change I.V. tubing, give site care, or rotate I.V. sites every 24 to 48 hours or according to hospital policy. • Encourage the patient to cough and deep-breathe at least every 4 hours after surgery. • Provide tissues and disposal bag for expectorated sputum. • Help the patient turn every 2 hours, if needed. Provide skin care where necessary. • Use sterile water to humidify oxygen. • Ensure adequate nutritional and fluid intake. • Teach the patient and his family how to recognize the signs of infection and about ways to avoid infection.	• Discuss with the patient and his family the importance of remaining infection-free. • Reinforce patient's treatment and care plan. • Advise patient when to seek medical care. • Arrange for follow-up care as needed.

in adult human blood. (For more information, see *Immune globulin: Protection against infection,* page 102.)

Immunoglobulin replacement therapy may benefit patients with these immunodeficiencies:

- agammaglobulinemia
- X-linked immunodeficiency with hyper-IgM
- antibody-mediated deficiency with near-normal immunoglobulin levels
- Wiskott-Aldrich syndrome
- severe combined immunodeficiency disease.

In other immunodeficiencies, immunoglobulin replacement therapy is usually contraindicated. For instance, infants with transient hy-

Continued on page 102

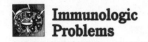

Primary and Secondary Immunodeficiency

Immune globulin: Protection against infection

Immune globulin (also known as gamma globulin or immune serum globulin) refers to a sterile, nonpyogenic globulin solution containing many antibodies normally found in an adult's blood. Manufacturers prepare immune globulin by cold alcohol fractionation of plasma pooled from the venous blood of 1,000 or more individuals. Depending on the preparation used, the resulting substance can be administered either I.M. or I.V.

To protect patients receiving any type of immune globulin, manufacturers must test all donated plasma for hepatitis B surface antigen and for antibodies to human immunodeficiency virus (HIV). Most likely, all immune globulin produced since April 1985 is free of HIV, because the manufacturing process includes purification steps highly effective in removing or inactivating the virus.

Doctors use immune globulin as replacement therapy in immunodeficiency disorders resulting from defective antibody synthesis. Immune globulin may also provide passive immunity in susceptible individuals exposed to hepatitis A and B, measles, rubella, varicella, or other infection. Other uses include the treatment of idiopathic thrombocytopenia purpura.

Immune globulin I.M.

Expect to administer immune globulin I.M. (IGIM) in patients with IgG deficiency and other antibody deficiency disorders to help prevent infection. IGIM shouldn't be used in selective IgA deficiency disorder. Trade names include Gamastan, Gammar, and Immuglobin.

Inject IGIM into the deltoid muscle or the anterolateral aspect of the thigh. To avoid injury to the sciatic nerves, avoid injections into the gluteal muscle's upper, outer quadrant unless administering a large volume to an adult or dividing a large dose into multiple injections. In neonates and small children, use only the anterolateral aspect of the thigh for I.M. injection.

As ordered, give 1.2 ml/kg initially, followed by a maintenance dose of 0.6 ml/kg (at least 100 mg/kg) once every 2 to 4 weeks; some patients may need more frequent injections. A single dose shouldn't exceed 50 ml in adults, 30 ml in infants and small children.

After administration, muscle stiffness, pain, and tenderness usually occur at the injection site and persist for several hours. Local inflammation, urticaria, angioedema, headache, malaise, fever, arthralgia, and nephrotic syndrome may also occur.

Immune globulin I.V.

Expect to administer immune globulin I.V. (IGIV) mainly as maintenance therapy for patients unable to produce sufficient amounts of IgG antibodies. You may also administer it to promote passive immunity when patients have congenital agammaglobulinemia, common variable hypogammaglobulinemia, X-linked immunodeficiency with hyper-IgM, or combined immunodeficiency disorders. IGIV shouldn't be used for patients with selective IgA deficiency disorder. Trade names include Gammagard, Gamimune N, and Sandoglobulin.

Always administer IGIV through separate tubing; never mix it with other drugs or I.V. fluids. Dosage varies with the preparation used.

If you're using *Gammagard,* start the infusion within 2 hours of reconstitution. Infuse at a rate of 0.5 ml/kg/hour and, if no adverse reactions occur, gradually increase to a maximum of 4 ml/kg/hr. For replacement therapy, infuse 200 to 400 mg/kg once monthly.

If you're using *Gamimune N,* start with 0.01 to 0.02 ml/kg/minute for 30 minutes. If no adverse reactions occur, gradually increase to a maximum of 0.08 ml/kg/minute. For replacement therapy, infuse 100 to 200 mg/kg or 2 to 4 ml/kg once monthly. If the patient has a poor response or an insufficient IgG level, increase up to 400 mg/kg (or 8 ml/kg) or give the usual dose more frequently, as ordered.

If you're using *Sandoglobulin* for a patient with agammaglobulinemia or hypogammaglobulinemia, start with an initial dose of 30 mg/ml followed by an infusion of 0.5 to 1.0 ml/minute. After 15 to 30 minutes, increase up to 2.5 ml/minute, if needed. After the initial dose, use a solution containing 60 mg/ml if necessary. For replacement therapy, infuse 200 mg/kg once monthly. If the patient has a poor response or an insufficient IgG level, increase up to a maximum of 300 mg/kg or give the usual dose more frequently, as ordered.

Adverse reactions to IGIV occur in 10% of patients or fewer. Patients especially at risk for systemic adverse effects include those with agammaglobulinemia or hypogammaglobulinemia, those who have never received IGIV, and those who have received the drug during the preceding 8 weeks. Most reactions seem to hinge more on the rate of administration than on the dose. To relieve an adverse reaction, decrease the flow rate or stop the infusion temporarily, as ordered.

Adverse reactions to IGIV include pain in the chest, hip, or back; nausea and vomiting; fever and chills; malaise; fatigue; faintness; headache; chest tightness; and dyspnea. Mild diuresis may follow Gamimune N infusion because the drug contains maltose as a stabilizing agent.

Occasionally, IGIV causes a precipitous fall in blood pressure and signs and symptoms of anaphylaxis, even in patients without a history of sensitivity to immune globulin. These reactions usually appear 30 to 60 minutes after the infusion starts; as ordered, temporarily stop the infusion until symptoms have subsided. The reaction seems linked to the rate of administration; administering more than 1 ml/min of Sandoglobulin to patients who have agammaglobulinemia or hypogammaglobulinemia who are receiving the drug for the first time or who have received the drug within the preceding 8 weeks increases the risk of reaction.

Primary immunodeficiency disorders—*continued*

pogammaglobulinemia do not receive immune globulin therapy because it could suppress their innate capacity to form antibodies. Patients with selective IgA deficiency also do not receive this treatment, nor do patients with IgG subclass deficiency.

To combat severe cell-mediated deficiency, the doctor may perform a tissue transplant. MHC-compatible bone marrow and fetal thymic

Primary and Secondary Immunodeficiency

tissue have been successfully transplanted. Graft-versus-host (GVH) disease poses the greatest risk to recipients of bone marrow or fetal tissue transplants. Recently developed techniques to deplete all post-thymic T cells from donor bone marrow now allow safe haploidentical (half-matched) marrow transplants. (For information on bone marrow transplantation, see chapter 6.)

Patients with less severe forms of cell-mediated deficiency face a greater risk of GVH disease. Even those who receive immunosuppressive drugs before transplantation will likely resist engraftment. Recently, however, several patients with Wiskott-Aldrich syndrome and other partial cell-mediated immunodeficiencies have successfully received bone marrow (usually HLA-identical) transplants after immunosuppression with anti-LFA-1 antibody.

Preventing infection. Because immunosuppressed patients are susceptible to infection, you'll need to take preventive measures. Perform all procedures with extreme care. Wash your hands frequently and thoroughly. Use aseptic technique when caring for sites where infectious organisms could enter, such as entrance sites for catheters, central or peripheral lines, or endotracheal tubes. If you're responsible for nursing assignments, arrange for immunodeficient patients to receive care first to avoid cross-contamination.

Remember that the skin is the only intact defense left in many immunosuppressed patients. Observe pressure areas closely for signs of infection or skin breakdown. Turn immobile patients every hour. Perform passive range-of-motion exercises or encourage active range-of-motion exercises. Keep the skin well lubricated to prevent cracks caused by dryness. Avoid prolonged contact with wetness, which macerates skin.

Have the patient perform coughing and deep-breathing exercises every 4 to 6 hours. These exercises, along with postural drainage, help prevent respiratory infection. Be sure to assess respiratory status frequently to spot infection early.

Avoid administering live virus vaccines (such as oral polio, measles, or rubella vaccines) to immunosuppressed patients, their siblings, or other household members. Vaccination with a live virus or exposure to persons vaccinated with them can cause severe infection or even death among immunosuppressed patients.

Providing nutrition. A high-protein, high-calorie diet will bolster the immune system; conversely, poor nutrition increases the risk of illness. Carefully assess your patient's nutritional and fluid status and take steps to maintain or improve it as needed.

Giving psychological support. Begin with a holistic assessment of the psychological impact of the immunodeficiency disorder and hospitalization on the patient and his family. Then employ appropriate nursing measures to lessen anxiety and enhance comfort. Be sure to provide ongoing emotional support, keeping in mind the numerous psychological hardships that accompany a life-threatening disease, repeated hospitalizations, and high-risk therapy:

- The patient is constantly reminded of his critical illness by medical and nursing activities, such as bone marrow transplants, use of

Continued on page 104

Primary and Secondary Immunodeficiency

Primary immunodeficiency disorders—*continued*

life-sustaining equipment, and intrusive procedures.
- If placed in reverse isolation or a bone marrow transplant unit, the patient may suffer from sensory deprivation and lack of physical contact. The patient may experience hallucinations, sleep disorders, or behavioral disorders as well as loneliness and depersonalization.
- The patient may develop profound feelings of helplessness, sadness, resentment, or anxiety.
- The patient may experience forced dependency; loss of control; or drastic changes in his body image, self-concept, and function.
- The patient's distress will, in turn, affect his family and, to a lesser extent, his social support group.

To ease the patient's psychological distress, try to strengthen his control over his circumstances. Develop a sense for his character, life-style, and aspirations. Emphasize his individuality and reinforce his coping mechanisms. Reassure him that someone cares about him and his reaction to illness. Encourage family, friends, staff, and other patients to offer support. Realistically discuss the patient's plans and rectify any misconceptions that he or his family may have about the disease, treatment, and plan of care.

Evaluation
Base your evaluation on the expected outcomes listed on the nursing care plan. To determine if the patient has improved, ask yourself these questions:
- Does the patient show any signs of infection?
- Does he know how to prevent infection?
- Can the patient, a family member, or both recognize the signs of infection?
- Does he understand the importance of preventing infection?

The answers to these questions will help you evaluate your patient's status and the effectiveness of his care. Keep in mind that these questions stem from the sample nursing care plan on page 101. Your questions may differ.

Selected primary immunodeficiency disorders

Primary immunodeficiency disorders may fall into one of five classes:
- antibody-mediated (B-cell) deficiency
- cell-mediated (T-cell) deficiency
- combined antibody- and cell-mediated deficiency
- phagocytic dysfunction
- complement deficiency.

For a classification of selected primary immunodeficiency disorders, see *Classifying immunodeficiencies*.

Antibody-mediated immunodeficiency disorders
Patients affected with these disorders may lack any or all of the immunoglobulin classes. The degree of antibody-mediated deficiency usually determines the severity of symptoms.

Primary and Secondary Immunodeficiency

Classifying immunodeficiencies

Immunodeficiencies can be classified into five groups: antibody-mediated (B-cell) disorders, cell-mediated (T-cell) disorders, combined antibody- and cell-mediated disorders, phagocytic deficiency disorders, and complement deficiency disorders.

Antibody-mediated immunodeficiency disorders	Cell-mediated immunodeficiency disorders	Combined antibody- and cell-mediated disorders	Phagocytic immunodeficiency disorders	Complement deficiency disorders
• B-cell immunodeficiency associated with 5′-nucleotidase deficiency • B-cell immunodeficiency related to drugs or protein loss • Selective IgA deficiency • Selective IgM deficiency • Selective deficiency of IgG subclasses • Immunodeficiency with hyper-IgM • Common, variable, unclassifiable immunodeficiency • Transient hypogammaglobulinemia of infancy • X-linked hypogammaglobulinemia • X-linked lymphoproliferative disease	• Chronic mucocutaneous candidiasis • DiGeorge syndrome (congenital thymic aplasia) • T-cell deficiency associated with absent Class I MHC antigens • T-cell deficiency associated with absent membrane glycoprotein • T-cell deficiency associated with purine-nucleoside phosphorylase deficiency	• Acquired immunodeficiency syndrome • Graft-versus-host disease • Severe combined immunodeficiency disease • Nezelof's syndrome • Immunodeficiency with ataxia-telangiectasia • Wiskott-Aldrich syndrome • Episodic lymphopenia with lymphotoxin • Immunodeficiency with thymoma • Immunodeficiency with short-limbed dwarfism • Immunodeficiency with adenosine deaminase deficiency	• Chronic granulomatous disease • Chédiak-Higashi syndrome • Job's syndrome • Lazy leukocyte syndrome • Glucose-6-phosphate dehydrogenase deficiency • Myeloperoxidase deficiency • Tuftsin deficiency • Elevated IgE, defective chemotaxis, eczema, and recurrent infections	• C1q, C1r, and C1s deficiency • C2 deficiency • C3 deficiency, types I and II • C4 deficiency • C5 deficiency or dysfunction • C6 deficiency • C7 deficiency • C8 deficiency • C9 deficiency

Antibody-mediated immunodeficiency disorders include:

- X-linked infantile hypogammaglobulinemia
- common variable immunodeficiency
- selective IgA deficiency
- transient hypogammaglobulinemia of infancy
- Duncan's syndrome
- immunodeficiency with hyper-IgM
- selective IgM deficiency
- selective deficiency of IgG subclasses.

Diagnostic tests. The following tests help to determine antibody-mediated immunodeficiency disorders:

- immunoelectrophoresis, to presumptively diagnose hypogammaglobulinemia or to evaluate for paraproteins
- radial immunodiffusion, to determine IgG, IgM, IgA, and IgD levels
- radioimmunoassay, to determine IgE levels
- Schick test, to evaluate IgG function
- isohemagglutinin titer, to evaluate IgM function
- specific antibody response, to evaluate immunoglobulin function
- B-cell count, to measure circulating B cells
- in vitro immunoglobulin synthesis, to determine T-helper and T-suppressor cell function in hypogammaglobulinemia.

Continued on page 106

Primary and Secondary Immunodeficiency

Transient hypogammaglobulinemia of infancy

A disease of unknown cause, transient hypogammaglobulinemia interrupts normal immunologic development, rendering some infants unusually susceptible to infection during early life. Normally, beginning at 16 weeks of gestation, the mother passively transfers IgG to her infant. (IgA, IgM, IgD, and IgE usually don't cross the placenta.) At birth, the infant's serum IgG level probably exceeds that of its mother. At age 4 to 5 months, serum IgG begins to decline gradually and serum IgM and IgA begin to rise gradually; IgM usually rises more rapidly than IgA. Serum IgG reaches its lowest level (about 350 mg/dl) around age 5 to 6 months, inducing physiologic hypogammaglobulinemia. Many normal infants suffer recurrent respiratory tract infections at this stage of life.

In transient hypogammaglobulinemia of infancy, the period when IgG levels are decreased lengthens, sometimes to as long as 2 years. Occasionally, such an infant requires immune globulin therapy. The patient should receive no routine immunizations during the period of transient hypogammaglobulinemia. Once his immune system becomes established, he can receive routine immunizations.

Duncan's syndrome

Also known as X-linked lymphoproliferative syndrome, Duncan's syndrome is a recessive trait characterized by an impaired immune response to Epstein-Barr virus (EBV). Agranulocytosis or cardiovascular or CNS birth defects may accompany the syndrome.

Patients appear healthy until they contract infectious mononucleosis. Many die as a result of overwhelming EBV-induced B-cell proliferation during mononucleosis. Those who survive the primary infection tend to develop hypogammaglobulinemia, B-cell lymphomas, or both.

Diagnostic tests show impaired production of antibodies to the EBV nuclear antigen. Titers of antibodies to the viral capsid antigen range from zero to markedly elevated levels.

Primary immunodeficiency disorders—*continued*

X-linked infantile hypogammaglobulinemia. Also called Bruton's disease, X-linked infantile hypogammaglobulinemia is characterized by deficiency or absence of all five immunoglobulin classes. B-cell precursors may not be present, resulting in complete absence of plasma cells and peripheral blood B cells.

Assessment. This disease strikes male infants, usually by the time they reach 5 to 6 months old. The decline of transplacentally acquired maternal immunoglobulin and the infant's increasing exposure to pathogens lead to the onset of symptoms. Assess the patient for severe chronic bacterial infections, most commonly from *Streptococcus pneumoniae* and *Haemophilus influenzae.* Initial symptoms include:

- bacterial otitis media
- bronchitis
- dermatitis
- eczematoid skin infections
- meningitis
- pneumonia.

The patient may develop arthritis, malabsorption, hepatitis, or polio. Chronic respiratory or GI problems may result from lack of secretory IgA. Occasionally, symptoms do not appear until early childhood; such patients may suffer chronic conjunctivitis, caries, or malabsorption.

Suspect X-linked infantile hypogammaglobulinemia if:

- infections fail to respond completely or promptly to appropriate antibiotic therapy
- the patient suffers bouts of illness without intervening periods of good health
- lymphadenopathy or splenomegaly do not accompany the repeated infections.

Diagnostic tests confirm the disorder, revealing an absence or marked deficiency of all immunoglobulin classes. Although immunoelectrophoresis may establish a diagnosis, most doctors perform specific quantitation of immunoglobulins, especially during early infancy. Test results show:

- total serum immunoglobulin level below 250 mg/dl
- serum IgG level usually below 200 mg/dl
- IgA, IgD, and IgE levels extremely low or absent.

Rarely, the doctor may perform intestinal biopsy to determine whether plasma cells are absent. The biopsy would show an absence of plasma cells in the lamina propria of the gut. Studies of peripheral blood lymphocytes may show an absence of circulating B cells.

Intervention. Immune globulin therapy usually controls X-linked infantile hypogammaglobulinemia, but unresponsive patients may require additional therapy. Because commercial immune globulin contains primarily IgG and little IgM or IgA, some doctors consider infusions of fresh-frozen plasma beneficial. The patient may undergo antibiotic therapy. To prevent fatal infections, the patient should receive no live virus vaccines.

Primary and Secondary Immunodeficiency

Immunodeficiency with hyper-IgM

A rare disorder of unknown cause, this immunodeficiency is characterized by increased IgM levels and depressed IgG and IgA levels. Most commonly, the disorder seems to be inherited as an X-linked trait.

The disorder causes recurrent pyogenic infections, such as otitis media, pneumonia, and septicemia. It may also cause recurrent neutropenia, hemolytic anemia, or aplastic anemia. What's more, it may increase the risk of an infiltrating cancer of IgM-producing cells.

Diagnostic tests may show:
- sharply increased serum IgM levels (150 to 1,000 mg/dl) with low or absent serum IgG and IgA levels
- elevated isohemagglutinin titers with possible antibody formation following immunization.

Treatment is similar to that given for infantile X-linked hypogammaglobulinemia.

Selective IgM deficiency

This rare deficiency is characterized by absence of IgM, but normal levels of other immunoglobulins. Of unknown cause, the deficiency increases susceptibility to autoimmune disease and to overwhelming infection with such polysaccharide-containing organisms as pneumococci and *Haemophilus influenzae.* Affected patients may complain of chronic dermatitis, diarrhea, and recurrent respiratory infections.

Expect to provide appropriate antibiotic therapy to treat infection. The doctor may order immune globulin therapy for patients unable to form antibodies to specific antigens.

Common variable immunodeficiency. Also called acquired hypogammaglobulinemia, common variable immunodeficiency shares the signs and symptoms of X-linked hypogammaglobulinemia but strikes males and females of all ages. The cause of this immunodeficiency isn't currently known, but most patients have an intrinsic B-cell defect.

Assessment. Symptoms usually arise between ages 15 and 35, with patients showing heightened susceptibility to autoimmune disorders, such as systemic lupus erythematosus (SLE), and to pyogenic infections. Commonly, patients show signs of chronic recurrent sinopulmonary infections and chronic bacterial conjunctivitis, and may also have marked lymphadenopathy and splenomegaly.

Diagnostic tests usually show:
- total serum immunoglobulin level below 300 mg/dl
- serum IgG level below 250 mg/dl
- normal amounts of peripheral blood B lymphocytes
- variable IgM and IgA levels or even absence of these immunoglobulins
- low or absent titers of isohemagglutinins.

The Schick test may demonstrate lack of normal antibody response. In patients with borderline immunoglobulin levels, such a response usually establishes the diagnosis.

Intervention. Provide care similar to that for infantile X-linked hypogammaglobulinemia. As ordered, give 20 to 40 ml of immune globulin I.M. monthly, 1 to 2 units of fresh-frozen plasma I.V. monthly, and antibiotics continuously in ordered combinations. Because large I.M. injections of immune globulin may cause considerable pain, the doctor may instead order monthly I.V. injections of 100 to 400 mg/kg. During acute illness, expect to administer the I.V. dosage weekly or even daily. Treat associated disorders appropriately.

Patients with common variable immunodeficiency may live to age 70 or 80. They're most likely to suffer chronic lung disease and face an increased risk of such malignancies as leukemia, lymphoma, and gastric carcinoma. Patients who develop acquired T-cell deficiencies experience increasing difficulty with infections characteristic of both T-cell and B-cell deficiencies.

Selective IgA deficiency. The most common primary immunodeficiency disorder, selective IgA deficiency has no known cause. It may result from arrested B-cell development. However, patients have normal levels of circulating IgA, suggesting reduced IgA synthesis or release. IgA deficiency may also result from arrested development of immunoglobulin-producing cells during the normal sequential development of IgM to IgG. Deficient secretory IgA may lead to increased or prolonged exposure to a spectrum of microbes and nonreplicating antigens, resulting in diseases associated with the disorder (such as autoimmune disease and cancer). Researchers recently discovered an increased prevalence of HLA-A1, HLA-A2, HLA-B8, and HLA-Dw3 in patients with IgA deficiency and autoimmune disease.

Continued on page 108

Primary and Secondary Immunodeficiency

Selective deficiency of IgG subclasses

This deficiency is characterized by normal levels of IgM and IgA but reduced levels of various combinations of IgG_1, IgG_2, IgG_3, and IgG_4. Depending on the disorder's severity, total serum IgG may be normal or reduced. Affected patients may or may not produce antibodies after immunization.

Selective IgG subclass deficiency heightens susceptibility to repeated pyogenic respiratory infections caused by pneumococci, *Haemophilus influenzae,* and *Staphylococcus aureus.* Treatment usually includes antibiotics and immune globulin.

Primary immunodeficiency disorders—*continued*

Assessment. Obtain a family health history. Find out if the patient's family has a history of such immunodeficiency disorders as hypogammaglobulinemia. If so, the patient has a greater than average likelihood of acquiring selective IgA deficiency. Find out if the patient's receiving phenytoin or penicillamine. These drugs may cause acquired IgA deficiency. Once drug therapy ends, the IgA level may return to normal.

Be alert for signs of recurrent viral or bacterial sinopulmonary infections, allergy, celiac disease, ulcerative colitis, and regional enteritis. Assess for an autoimmune disorder, such as SLE, rheumatoid arthritis, dermatomyositis, pernicious anemia, thyroiditis, Coombs-positive hemolytic anemia, Sjögren's syndrome, or chronic active hepatitis. Selective IgA deficiency may also lead to reticulum cell sarcoma, squamous cell carcinoma of the esophagus and lung, and thymoma.

IgA-deficient patients who produce normal amounts of IgG and IgM may be asymptomatic. However, long-term follow-up indicates that these patients still risk developing significant disease.

Diagnostic tests reveal a serum IgA level under 5 mg/dl, with normal or increased IgG, IgM, IgD, and IgE. Typically, secretory IgA is absent in both serum and secretions, while other normal secretory components are present. Autoantibody formation increases, including antibodies directed against IgG, IgM, and IgA. Serum B-cell count remains normal. Other laboratory abnormalities are characteristic of the associated diseases.

Intervention. The doctor will not use immune globulin to replace deficient IgA. Patients with selective IgA deficiency can form normal levels of antibodies to other immunoglobulin classes and may recognize injected IgA as foreign. So administering immune globulin increases the patient's risk of developing anti-IgA antibodies and subsequent anaphylactic transfusion reaction.

Antimicrobial agents to combat specific infections constitute the only treatment currently available against selective IgA deficiency. Carefully monitor patients for infection and administer appropriate antibiotics. To avoid permanent pulmonary complications, expect to treat recurrent sinopulmonary infections aggressively with broad-spectrum antibiotics. Patients who also have autoimmune disorders such as SLE, rheumatoid arthritis, and celiac disease require the usual therapy for these disorders.

If the patient with selective IgA deficiency requires a blood transfusion, minimize the risk of a reaction by:
- using washed packed red blood cells
- using donor blood from a matched IgA-deficient person
- freezing the patient's own blood for future use.

Cell-mediated immunodeficiency disorders

Cell-mediated immunodeficiency disorders are characterized by defective T-cell immunity. Most patients have abnormalities of B-cell immunity as well. Some have normal immunoglobulin levels but

Primary and Secondary Immunodeficiency

Facial features of DiGeorge syndrome

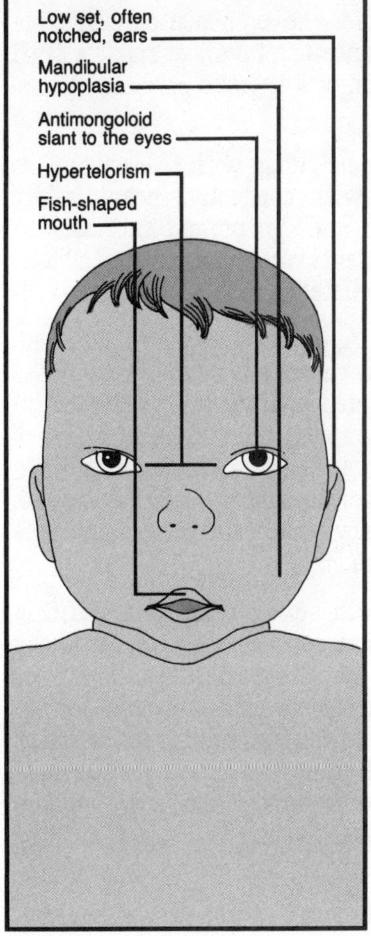

fail to produce specific antibodies after immunization. The condition leads to increased susceptibility to acute or chronic infections. Cell-mediated immunodeficiency disorders include DiGeorge syndrome and chronic mucocutaneous candidiasis.

Diagnostic tests. Various tests help detect cell-mediated immunodeficiency disorders, including:
- white blood cell (WBC) count
- delayed hypersensitivity skin test, to evaluate specific immunity to antigens
- lymphocyte response to mitogens, antigens, and allogeneic cells (mixed lymphocyte culture), to evaluate T-cell function
- T-cell rosettes (E rosettes), to determine the number of circulating T cells
- monoclonal antibody to T cells and T-cell subsets, to determine total number of T cells and T-cell subsets, such as helper and suppressor cells
- cytokine production, to provide an index of the function of mononuclear cell subsets
- T-cell count.

DiGeorge syndrome. Also called congenital thymic aplasia or hypoplasia, DiGeorge syndrome probably results from abnormal embryologic development at about 12 weeks of gestation. Some patients have no thymus; others have an abnormally located or extremely small one. Because a fetal thymus transplant may restore T-cell immunity, early diagnosis is critical.

Assessment. Unlike most other immunodeficiencies, DiGeorge syndrome produces symptoms that are apparent at birth. Look for abnormal facies with low-set ears, fish-shaped mouth, hypertelorism, notched ear pinnae, micrognathia, short philtrum of the upper lip, mandibular hypoplasia, and an antimongoloid slant to the eyes. (See *Facial features of DiGeorge syndrome*.) Hypoparathyroidism commonly leads to hypocalcemia in the first 24 hours of life. Suspect DiGeorge syndrome if hypocalcemia resists standard therapy. Congenital heart defects, including interruption of the aortic arch, septal defects, patent ductus arteriosus, and truncus arteriosus, may accompany other symptoms. Renal abnormalities may be present as well.

An infant who survives the immediate neonatal period may develop recurrent or chronic viral, bacterial, fungal, or protozoal infections. Be alert for signs of pneumonia, chronic candidal infection of the mucous membranes, diarrhea, and failure to thrive.

Tests demonstrating defective T-cell immunity confirm DiGeorge syndrome. The WBC count is usually low but may be normal or elevated. A lateral X-ray view of the anterior mediastinum may reveal absence of the thymic shadow, indicating failure of normal development. Low serum calcium levels may accompany elevated serum phosphorus levels and absence of parathyroid hormone, indicating hypoparathyroidism.

Intervention. A fetal thymus transplant should be performed as quickly as possible to restore cell-mediated immunity. The new thymus may be implanted locally in the *rectus abdominis* muscle or

Continued on page 110

Primary and Secondary Immunodeficiency

Primary immunodeficiency disorders—*continued*

in a Millipore chamber. Alternately, the thymus may be minced and injected intraperitoneally. Transplanted glands should be no older than 14 weeks gestation; otherwise, the presence of viable immunocompetent lymphocytes will place the infant at risk for GVH disease. Thymosin may also be given or a thymus epithelial transplant performed.

Give vitamin D or parathyroid hormone along with oral calcium to control hypocalcemia. The infant with congestive heart failure caused by congenital defect should undergo prompt surgical correction. To prevent GVH disease, patients who must undergo a blood transfusion should receive only irradiated blood.

Chronic mucocutaneous candidiasis. Apparently inherited as an autosomal recessive trait, chronic mucocutaneous candidiasis results from a selective defect in cell-mediated immunity. The disease increases susceptibility to chronic candidal infection, especially of the skin, nails, and mucous membranes. In some patients, autoantibodies develop, attack the endocrine system, and induce idiopathic endocrinopathy. B-cell immunity remains intact and produces a normal antibody response to *Candida*.

Assessment. This disease strikes both sexes, usually in the first year of life, although onset may occur as late as the teens. Check for signs of localized infection in the mucous membranes, skin, nails and, in older women, the vagina. In severe forms, observe for the "stocking glove" pattern of skin infection and for the formation of granulomatous lesions. Infection often spreads from the perineal and circumoral areas to the extremities, scalp, and face. Candidal laryngitis and esophagitis are common; systemic candidal infection is rare.

Also be alert for the gradual development of potentially fatal endocrine dysfunction. Idiopathic endocrinopathy may occur before candidal infection or several years afterward. The most common endocrine effects are hypoparathyroidism and Addison's disease.

Diagnostic tests consistently reveal a defect in T-cell immunity. The degree of this defect will vary. At minimum, the patient will not respond to a delayed hypersensitivity skin test for *Candida* antigen. The WBC count tends to be normal.

Intervention. Be prepared for difficulties when treating chronic candidal infection of the skin and mucous membranes. Topical antifungal drugs may not help. However, patients may benefit from local or I.V. miconazole, oral clotrimazole, and oral ketoconazole. I.V. administration of amphotericin B may also help, but renal toxicity limits the drug's usefulness. However, it may be combined with subcutaneous transfer factor therapy. Before or during amphotericin therapy (or both), expect to administer transfer factor from donors who react positively to *Candida* skin tests. No treatment can stop development of idiopathic endocrinopathy.

Expect frequent illness in patients who live past age 20 or 30. Patients who suffer severe candidal infection of the mucous mem-

Primary and Secondary Immunodeficiency

Immunodeficiency with short-limbed dwarfism

Immunodeficiency is associated with three types of short-limbed dwarfism. Each of these types has distinctive symptoms, but all affected patients display these characteristics:
• short, pudgy limbs and hands
• normal-sized head, which distinguishes this disorder from achondroplasia
• extra skin folds around the neck
• large limb joints during infancy.

Patients with Type I short-limbed dwarfism have no T-cell or B-cell immunity. Their symptoms resemble those of severe combined immunodeficiency disease, including susceptibility to viral, bacterial, fungal, and protozoal infection. Patients rarely survive beyond age 1.

Patients with Type II short-limbed dwarfism have deficient T-cell immunity and normal B-cell immunity. Diagnosis depends on delayed hypersensitivity skin tests and the responsiveness of peripheral blood lymphocytes. These patients may develop cartilage-hair hypoplasia (characterized by light, thin, sparse hair), a malabsorption-like syndrome, recurrent sinopulmonary infections, progressive vaccinia, or fatal varicella.

Patients with Type III short-limbed dwarfism have deficient B-cell immunity and normal T-cell immunity. They may experience such recurrent pyogenic infections as meningitis, otitis media, pneumonia, and sepsis.

Treatment of the three types of short-limbed dwarfism depends upon the associated immunodeficiency.

branes and skin may become psychologically upset and need strong emotional support.

Combined antibody- and cell-mediated immunodeficiency disorders
Typically, combined antibody- and cell-mediated immunodeficiency disorders produce symptoms early in infancy and heighten susceptibility to a wide range of infections. The severity of these disorders varies; patients may retain partial T-cell and B-cell immunity, or completely lack both mechanisms of host defense. Immunotherapy is frequently difficult and often unavailable.

Combined immunodeficiency disorders stem from a variety of causes and include:
• severe combined immunodeficiency disease
• Nezelof's syndrome
• ataxia-telangiectasia
• Wiskott-Aldrich syndrome
• immunodeficiency with thymoma
• immunodeficiency with short-limbed dwarfism
• enzyme-related immunodeficiencies
• cell membrane abnormalities
• GVH disease (see Chapter 6)
• acquired immunodeficiency syndrome (see Chapter 4).

Diagnostic tests. The patient will undergo tests for evaluating both T-cell and B-cell immunity. An analysis of red and white blood cell enzymes (adenosine deaminase and nucleoside phosphorylase) may also help to properly classify a disorder.

Severe combined immunodeficiency disease (SCID). The most severe immunodeficiency disorder, SCID indicates a complete lack of both T-cell and B-cell immunity. Patients succumb to virtually any type of microbial infection. Few survive past age 1.

SCID has two types: X-linked lymphopenic agammaglobulinemia, which is transmitted as a recessive trait, and Swiss-type lymphopenic agammaglobulinemia, which is an autosomal recessive trait. All SCID disorders share an apparent congenital absence of adaptive immune function and a great diversity of genetic, enzymatic, hematologic, and immunologic features. Their exact incidence isn't known.

Some immunologists say that SCID results from the failure of stem cells to differentiate into T cells and B cells. However, others argue that the defect originates in the failure of the thymus and bursal equivalent tissue to develop normally.

Assessment. When the patient reaches about 6 months of age, the following symptoms may develop:
• failure to thrive
• chronic diarrhea
• persistent oral candidiasis (thrush)
• pneumonia
• chronic otitis media
• dehydration

Continued on page 112

Primary and Secondary Immunodeficiency

Enzyme-related immunodeficiencies

Several immunodeficiencies are associated with a shortage of enzymes.

Adenosine deaminase and nucleoside phosphorylase deficiency	5′-nucleotidase deficiency	Transcobalamin II deficiency	Biotin-dependent carboxylase deficiency
These enzymes are necessary for purine catabolism. Deficiency may disturb T-cell and B-cell immunity, causing mild abnormalities to complete absence of immunity. Because the degree of combined immunodeficiency varies, you'll see inconsistent symptoms, differing age of onset, and variable response to treatment. Doctors may treat adenosine deaminase and nucleoside phosphorylase deficiency with bone marrow transplants, infusion of irradiated red blood cells (a source of the enzyme), thymosin therapy, or thymus transplantation.	Researchers have linked decreased activity of 5′-nucleotidase with acquired hypogammaglobulinemia, X-linked hypogammaglobulinemia, and selective IgA deficiency.	Transcobalamin is a vitamin B_{12}–binding protein needed to transport vitamin B_{12} into cells. Deficiency may cause granulocytopenia, hypogammaglobulinemia, lymphopenia, macrocytic anemia, severe intestinal malabsorption, and thrombocytopenia. Vitamin B_{12} therapy usually reverses the symptoms.	This disorder causes abnormalities in both B-cell and T-cell function. Its features include ataxia; alopecia; increased excretion of beta-hydroxypropionate, methylcitrate, beta-methylcrotonyl-glycine, and 3-beta-hydroxyisovalerate in the urine; infantile chronic mucocutaneous candidiasis; and intermittent lactic acidosis. Multiple biotin-dependent carboxylase deficiencies may lead to chronic mucocutaneous candidiasis with abnormal T-cell function or severe recurrent sepsis. Treatment with biotin can reduce abnormal metabolites in the urine and reverse alopecia, ataxia, and chronic candidiasis.

Primary immunodeficiency disorders—*continued*

- developmental retardation
- viral, bacterial, fungal, protozoal, and other infections, such as *Candida*, cytomegalovirus, and *Pneumocystis carinii* infection.

GVH disease may follow maternal infusion of cells during gestation or delivery, or infusions of viable cells during blood transfusion or immunotherapy.

The presence of maternal IgG makes diagnosis difficult during the infant's first 5 to 6 months of life. Tests of T-cell immunity may detect lymphopenia, absence of thymic shadow, depressed T cells, and lack of response to delayed hypersensitivity skin tests. Tests of B-cell immunity may detect hypogammaglobulinemia and decreased or absent numbers of circulating B cells. Also, some infants fail to show an antibody response after immunization. Additional tests may be necessary, depending on the infant's signs and symptoms.

Intervention. As ordered, provide prompt, aggressive therapy for infections. If you administer blood products, be sure they've been irradiated to eradicate potentially viable lymphocytes. Do not administer attenuated virus vaccines. Transplantation of histocompatible bone marrow is the definitive treatment. However, despite careful matching, the SCID patient risks GVH reaction. The doctor may also order administration of immune globulin.

In the absence of a histocompatible bone marrow donor, the doctor may perform a fetal liver or thymus transplant, a thymus epithelial transplant, or a combined fetal liver and thymus transplant.

Immunodeficiency with thymoma

In this disorder, a primary benign or malignant thymic tumor (thymoma) develops along with combined antibody- and cell-mediated immunodeficiency. Also called Good's syndrome, the disorder usually strikes patients over age 40 and men more often than women.

Recurrent infection, the most common complaint, may be accompanied by aplastic anemia, chronic diarrhea, dermatitis, septicemia, respiratory infection, and urinary tract infection. Diagnostic tests may reveal marked hypogammaglobulinemia and deficient cellular immunity. Patients with acquired hypogammaglobulinemia should have regular chest X-rays to help detect thymoma as early as possible.

Thymoma removal alone won't reverse the immunodeficiency; therapy aims to control the immunoglobulin deficiency as well. Immune globulin can help control recurrent infections, but prognosis is poor.

113 Immunodeficiency Disorders

Primary and Secondary Immunodeficiency

Immunodeficiency with cell membrane abnormalities

Some immunodeficiencies are related to deficiency of an essential cell membrane component.

Bare lymphocyte syndrome	LFA-1/Mac-1 glycoprotein deficiency	gpL-115 glycoprotein deficiency
Some patients with this syndrome remain healthy, while others develop aplastic anemia, chronic diarrhea, opportunistic or recurring infections, and varying degrees of immunodeficiency. Symptomatic patients are lymphopenic and display decreased T-cell levels and normal or elevated B-cell levels.	This disorder is characterized by delayed umbilical cord separation, granulocytosis, impaired inflammatory response, and recurring bacterial infection. Granulocytes and monocytes function abnormally, leading to decreased adherence and phagocytosis of opsonized particles and to decreased chemotaxis.	Patients with this disorder experience recurrent bacterial, protozoal, and viral infections. Diagnostic tests reveal normal serum immunoglobulin levels, a decreased lymphocytic response to mitogens and specific antigens, and a reduced number of lymphocytes.

Nezelof's syndrome. In this syndrome, cell-mediated immunodeficiency accompanies abnormal immunoglobulin synthesis. The syndrome consists of various disorders characterized by markedly deficient T-cell immunity and varying degrees of deficient B-cell immunity. These disorders probably don't share a single cause, although the pathology of Nezelof's syndrome indicates a defect in the thymus. The syndrome occurs sporadically in both males and females, with no apparent genetic pattern.

Assessment. Symptoms usually appear in infancy. The patient becomes susceptible to recurrent fungal, protozoal, viral, and bacterial infections. Signs and symptoms may include recurrent or chronic pulmonary infections, failure to thrive, oral or cutaneous candidiasis, chronic diarrhea, recurrent skin infections, gram-negative sepsis, urinary tract infections, severe progressive varicella, and marked lymphadenopathy and hepatosplenomegaly.

Diagnostic tests may show:
- abnormal T-cell immunity, with varying degrees of deficiency
- lymphopenia, although a normal WBC count is possible
- moderately to markedly decreased T cells
- absent to slightly depressed lymphocyte response to specific antigens
- absent to normal lymphocyte response to allogeneic cells
- abnormal B-cell immunity
- normal circulating B-cell levels, with possible variation in distribution among various types of surface immunoglobulin-bearing B cells
- absent or normal isohemagglutinin titers
- reactive or nonreactive Schick test.

Intervention. As ordered, provide aggressive treatment for infection, including continuous broad-spectrum antibiotic coverage. Even if immunoglobulin levels are normal, the doctor may administer immune globulin to patients who fail to show an antibody response after immunization. Surprisingly, histocompatible bone marrow transplantation rarely succeeds. Thymus transplantation or thymic factor therapy may restore T-cell immunity and partly restore B-cell immunity. The doctor may also order transfer factor therapy.

Continued on page 114

Primary and Secondary Immunodeficiency

Primary immunodeficiency disorders—*continued*

Do not administer attenuated virus vaccines. Before transfusion, make sure all blood products are irradiated.

Ataxia-telangiectasia. Transmitted as an autosomal recessive trait, ataxia-telangiectasia attacks the neurologic, vascular, endocrine, and immune systems. Its exact cause remains unknown, but the disorder may result from an abnormality in deoxyribonucleic acid (DNA) repair.

Assessment. Signs and symptoms may include ataxia, telangiectasis, recurrent sinopulmonary infection, and abnormalities in B-cell and T-cell immunity.

Symptoms of progressive cerebellar ataxia usually appear at age 9 months to 1 year, though onset may be delayed until age 4 to 6 years. Watch for the development of choreoathetoid movements, disconjugate gaze, and extrapyramidal and posterior column signs. With the passage of time, expect neurologic abnormalities to become more severe.

Oculocutaneous telangiectasia usually appears by age 2 but may not develop until age 8 or 9. Typically, lesions appear first in the bulbar conjunctiva and subsequently on the bridge of the nose, the ears, or in the antecubital fossae.

Signs of recurrent pulmonary infection may appear early in life or as late as age 10.

Most patients fail to develop secondary sexual characteristics at puberty and most appear to develop mental retardation. Immunodeficiency worsens with time. Patients face a great risk of lymphoreticular malignancies, including lymphoma and acute lymphocytic leukemia. At best, patients survive into their forties. Death usually follows the development of overwhelming infection or malignancy.

Diagnostic test results may show:
- abnormality in T-cell and B-cell immunity, in varying degrees
- deficient or absent IgA (occurs in more than 40% of patients)
- lymphopenia
- normal or decreased T cells
- low concentrations of IgE.

Other laboratory abnormalities relate to associated findings.

Intervention. To avoid permanent complications, treat recurrent sinopulmonary infections promptly. Some patients may benefit from continuous broad-spectrum antibiotic therapy. The doctor may also order transfer factor therapy, bone marrow transplantation, thymus transplantation, or thymic factor therapy. Intravenous immune globulin therapy may help reduce the number of infections in patients unable to form antibody.

Do not administer attenuated viral vaccines and administer only irradiated blood products, if needed.

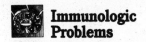

Primary and Secondary Immunodeficiency

Wiskott-Aldrich syndrome. This X-linked recessive immunodeficiency is characterized by a triad of symptoms: eczema, thrombocytopenic purpura with bleeding, and susceptibility to recurrent infection. The cause is uncertain, although some immunologists believe both the patient and carrier have abnormal platelets and macrophages.

Assessment. At birth, patients usually show signs of thrombocytopenia, with a decreased platelet count and severe bleeding. If the patient becomes infected, bleeding will increase. Check for signs of prolonged bleeding at the circumcision site. Bloody diarrhea is also common.

At about age 6 months, expect the patient to show signs of recurrent infection, most likely from capsular polysaccharide-type organisms such as *Pneumococcus, Meningococcus,* and *Haemophilus influenzae.* Patients may develop otitis media, pneumonia, meningitis, or sepsis.

As the child grows, bleeding episodes should become less severe, but susceptibility to infection increases and involves a widening variety of organisms. Patients face a high risk of recurrent viral infection, such as herpesvirus infection, and malignancies, such as lymphoreticular cancer.

By age 1, patients usually develop eczema, sometimes accompanied by other allergic disorders or secondary infection. Distribution of lesions is typical.

Diagnostic test results include:
- a platelet count ranging from 5,000 to 100,000/μl, indicating thrombocytopenia
- small platelets
- anemia, possibly indicated by positive Coombs' test
- normal IgG
- decreased IgM
- increased IgA and IgE
- low to absent isohemagglutinins
- normal numbers of B cells
- inability to respond to immunization with polysaccharide antigen
- intact T-cell immunity (may decline as the disease advances).

Intervention. Expect to treat infections promptly and aggressively with antibiotics. The use of corticosteroids to treat thrombocytopenia is contraindicated because the drug increases susceptibility to infection.

Expect difficulty in treating the immunodeficiency. Thrombocytopenia contraindicates I.M. immune globulin therapy because of potential bleeding at injection sites. The patient may, however, receive immune globulin I.V. or a bone marrow transplant to correct hematologic and immunologic abnormalities. Transfer factor has helped some patients; others have obtained passive protection from monthly transfusions of fresh-frozen plasma. The doctor may also perform a splenectomy to help increase the patient's platelet count, thereby reducing the risk of serious bleeding.

Continued on page 116

Primary and Secondary Immunodeficiency

Primary immunodeficiency disorders—*continued*

Phagocytic immunodeficiency disorders

These disorders produce symptoms ranging from mild recurrent skin conditions to fatal systemic infection. Although the patient is highly susceptible to bacteria and fungi, usually his immune system easily resists invasion from viral or protozoal organisms.

Extrinsic phagocytic disorders include:
- deficiencies of opsonins secondary to deficiencies of antibody and complement factors
- a decrease in phagocytic cells secondary to immunosuppressive therapy
- impaired phagocytic function secondary to corticosteroid therapy
- suppression of the number of circulating neutrophils by autoantibody directed specifically against neutrophil antigens
- complement deficiencies or abnormal complement components leading to abnormal neutrophil chemotaxis.

Intrinsic phagocytic disorders occur when enzymatic deficiencies impair the metabolic pathway for killing bacteria. Associated disorders include chronic granulomatous disease with NADPH or NADH oxidase deficiency, myeloperoxidase deficiency, and glucose-6-phosphate dehydrogenase deficiency.

Diagnostic studies. Tests to evaluate phagocytic dysfunction include:
- nitroblue tetrazolium (NBT) test, to diagnose chronic granulomatous disease and to detect carrier state
- intracellular killing curve test, to diagnose chronic granulomatous disease
- chemotaxis test, to detect disorders associated with frequent bacterial infection (does not provide a specific diagnosis)
- random migration, to test for lazy leukocyte syndrome by measuring nonchemotactic migration of leukocytes
- chemiluminescence, to test for chronic granulomatous disease and myeloperoxidase deficiency.

Chronic granulomatous disease. Inherited as an X-linked trait, chronic granulomatous disease leaves patients susceptible to infection from normally nonpathogenic and unusual organisms. In studying chronic granulomatous disease, scientists found an abnormality in the cytochrome of neutrophil cells. Patients with this defect are able to phagocytize but not kill catalase-positive bacteria such as *Staphylococcus aureus, Klebsiella aerobacter, Proteus, Serratia marcescens*, and such fungi as *Candida* and *Aspergillus*. Decreased intracellular killing of these bacteria and fungi brings on the signs and symptoms of the disease.

Assessment. Doctors can usually diagnose chronic granulomatous disease based on signs and symptoms that appear before age 2. These symptoms may include:
- lymphadenopathy
- hepatosplenomegaly
- chronic draining lymph nodes
- at least one episode of pneumonia
- prolonged fevers of unknown cause without localizing signs

Myeloperoxidase deficiency

Necessary for intracellular destruction of microorganisms, the enzyme myeloperoxidase is present in white blood cells and causes the green color of pus. Myeloperoxidase deficiency or absence, probably the most common primary neutrophil defect, increases susceptibility to candidal or staphylococcal infections.

Histochemical techniques help establish a diagnosis. Treatment includes antibiotics.

Other phagocytic cell disorders

Tuftsin deficiency
A phagocytosis-stimulating tetrapeptide, tuftsin is produced in the spleen and split from a parent immunoglobulin molecule called a leukokinin. A familial disorder, tuftsin deficiency leads to severe local and systemic infection. Complete lack of tuftsin may occur in splenectomy patients. No treatment is available and patients face an uncertain prognosis. Supportive therapy may include immune globulin.

Glucose-6-phosphate dehydrogenase (G6PD) deficiency
An X-linked trait, G6PD deficiency increases susceptibility to infection and produces symptoms resembling those of chronic granulomatous disease. Unlike chronic granulomatous disease, it affects both men and women and strikes later in life. The deficiency leads to hemolytic anemia.

Diagnostic studies reveal deficient G6PD in white blood cells. Abnormal nitroblue tetrazolium test results help to establish diagnosis. The treatment and prognosis for G6PD deficiency resemble that of chronic granulomatous disease.

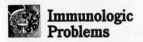

Primary and Secondary Immunodeficiency

Lazy leukocyte syndrome

A neutrophil defect characterized by defective chemotaxis, lazy leukocyte syndrome heightens susceptibility to recurrent severe infections, especially from such bacteria as *Staphylococcus*.

Neutropenia helps to establish the diagnosis, whereas a chemotactic assay shows reduced neutrophil mobility. Treatment calls for antibiotics.

Similar syndromes

Rarely causing systemic signs or inflammation, Job's syndrome produces persistent rhinorrhea, otitis media, eczematous skin lesions, and recurrent staphylococcal abscesses of the skin, lymph nodes, or subcutaneous tissue. Once thought to be a variant of chronic granulomatous disease, the syndrome closely resembles hyper-IgE syndrome, and shares similar laboratory features. In fact, the two conditions may be the same.

Hyper-IgE syndrome strikes both men and women and is characterized by early onset of eczema and recurrent bacterial infections in the form of abscesses. Infecting organisms may include *Staphylococcus aureus, Candida, Haemophilus influenzae, Streptococcus pneumoniae,* and group A streptococci. Abscesses may affect the skin, lungs, ears, sinuses, or eyes. Systemic infection may involve other areas.

Diagnostic tests may detect:
- IgE levels above 5,000 IU/ml
- reduced levels of T-suppressor cells with increased spontaneous IgE production
- eosinophilia
- defective chemotaxis
- diminished antibody response after immunization
- enhanced IgE antibody response to staphylococcal antigens.

Treatment includes antibiotics. The prognosis is uncertain; affected patients may survive to adulthood.

- infection subsequent to fever
- frequent chronic anemia, often exacerbated during fever
- rhinitis
- conjunctivitis
- dermatitis
- ulcerative stomatitis
- perianal abscess
- osteomyelitis
- chronic diarrhea with intermittent abdominal pains
- intestinal obstruction
- chronic and acute infection in lymph nodes, skin, lung, intestinal tract, liver, and bone.

The NBT test readily provides diagnostic information. The absence of nitroblue tetrazolium dye reduction indicates chronic granulomatous disease. Carriers may have normal or reduced NBT reduction.

The killing curves for infectious organisms will usually indicate little or no killing in a period of 2 hours. Hypergammaglobulinemia or an elevated WBC count—even in the absence of active infection—may occur. Detection of a normally nonpathogenic or unusual organism often provides a major clue to early diagnosis.

Intervention. Achieving long-term survival and lessening the severity of illness require aggressive therapy. Expect the doctor to order antibiotics to treat the infection. The doctor may also perform additional therapy, such as WBC infusions or bone marrow transplantation.

Chédiak-Higashi syndrome. This is a multisystem autosomal recessive syndrome. Neutrophils and monocytes become functionally defective, leading to impaired chemotactic response.

Assessment. Chédiak-Higashi syndrome is characterized by bacterial infections, hepatosplenomegaly, and CNS abnormalities. In addition, patients develop partial oculocutaneous albinism, and hair color may turn steel gray. Infection may follow exposure to a variety of bacterial organisms, but does not recur in all patients.

In many cases, the disease enters an accelerated phase. The patient develops an aggressive lymphoma-like disorder accompanied by hepatosplenomegaly, lymphadenopathy, pancytopenia, and sometimes lymphoreticular cancers.

Peripheral blood smears reveal giant cytoplasmic granular inclusions in WBCs and platelets. Other tests show:
- elevated Epstein-Barr virus antibody titers
- abnormal neutrophil chemotaxis
- decreased natural killer–cell activity
- abnormal intracellular killing of streptococci, pneumococci, and other organisms found in chronic granulomatous disease.

Intervention. Expect to provide specific antibiotic therapy to combat infecting organisms. Increasing susceptibility to infection and progressive neurologic deterioration make for a poor prognosis. Most patients die before age 5, although a few survive into their teens and twenties.

Continued on page 118

Primary and Secondary Immunodeficiency

Complement deficiency disorders

When an element of the complement system is deficient or absent, the following signs, symptoms, and associated disorders may occur.

Deficient or absent component	Signs, symptoms, and associated disorders
C1q	■ bacterial infection (usually gram-positive) ■ systemic lupus erythematosus–like (SLE-like) syndrome ■ associated with X-linked hypogammaglobulinemia and severe combined immunodeficiency disease
C1r C1s	■ SLE-like syndrome ■ bacterial infection (usually gram-positive)
C2	■ bacterial infection (usually gram-positive) ■ SLE-like syndrome ■ associated with hypogammaglobulinemia
C3	■ recurrent bacterial infection (usually gram-positive)
C4	■ bacterial infection (usually gram-positive) ■ SLE-like syndrome
C5	■ diarrhea ■ failure to thrive ■ recurrent bacterial infection, usually neisserial meningitis ■ seborrheic dermatitis
C6	■ recurrent disseminated gonococcal infection ■ recurrent neisserial meningitis infection
C7	■ disseminated gonococcal infection ■ recurrent neisserial meningitis infection ■ associated with ankylosing spondylitis, Raynaud's phenomenon, and telangiectasia
C8	■ recurrent disseminated gonococcal infection ■ recurrent neisserial meningitis infection
C9	■ usually no abnormal signs or symptoms

Primary immunodeficiency disorders—*continued*

Complement disorders

Several well-defined primary immunodeficiency disorders involve the complement system. In fact, immunologists have described genetically determined deficiencies for virtually all of the components of the complement system. (See *Complement deficiency disorders.*) For example, patients with C3, C5, C6, and C7 deficiencies are susceptible to infection. C3-deficient patients develop infections characteristic of antibody-mediated deficiency disorders. Patients with deficiencies in the terminal components usually incur meningococcal or gonococcal disorders. Many complement immunodeficiency disorders are associated with increased susceptibility to autoimmune disease. Supportive therapy may focus on treating infection with antibiotics or caring for associated disorders.

Hereditary angioedema. In hereditary angioedema, a deficiency in C1 esterase inhibitor leads to uncontrolled activation of the early components of the classical complement system. This causes the generation of a kininlike substance in the plasma, which in turn produces recurrent edema of the GI tract, skin, and upper respi-

Primary and Secondary Immunodeficiency

ratory mucosa (especially the larynx). The edema is nonpitting, nonpruritic, and unaccompanied by urticaria.

Assessment. Symptoms commonly include attacks of nausea, vomiting, abdominal pain, and potentially fatal edema of the upper airway. They may appear spontaneously or follow such trauma as dental work or emotional stress.

Diagnosis of hereditary angioedema is usually based on patient history. Tests to confirm diagnosis will show markedly diminished serum C4 levels, even when the patient has no symptoms. Levels of other complement components are usually normal. Tests to establish diagnosis include the immunoassay to measure C1 inactivator protein and the hemolytic assay to measure the protein's functional activity.

Intervention. Plasmin inhibitors, such as aminocaproic acid, may prevent or ameliorate attacks. To increase serum concentrations of C1 inactivator and C4, doctors may employ androgen therapy using methyltestosterone or attenuated sex hormones such as oxymetholone and danazol. This therapy helps prevent attacks as well. To ward off episodes induced by such trauma as dental surgery, doctors may attempt to supply the missing inactivator by administering fresh-frozen plasma.

Secondary immunodeficiency disorders

Unlike primary immunodeficiency disorders, secondary immunodeficiency disorders do not arise from intrinsic abnormalities in the development or function of T cells and B cells. Instead, such extrinsic factors as disease, therapy, or malnutrition cause an impaired immune response.

Secondary immunodeficiency disorders lead to increased susceptibility to opportunistic infection. Some patients experience only transient immunodeficiency and respond to adequate treatment of the primary cause. Others develop permanent immunodeficiency. Being able to recognize a state of secondary immunodeficiency will enable you to protect immunosuppressed patients from opportunistic infection.

Treatment depends upon the cause of the secondary immunodeficiency. (For information on the variety of disorders and therapeutic treatments, see *Mechanisms of selected secondary immunodeficiencies,* pages 120 and 121.)

Continued on page 121

Primary and Secondary Immunodeficiency

Mechanisms of selected secondary immunodeficiencies

	CELL-MEDIATED IMMUNITY	HUMORAL IMMUNITY		NONSPECIFIC IMMUNITY
Cause	**Effect on T cells**	**Effect on B cells**	**Effect on complement**	**Effect on phagocytosis**
INFECTION				
Acute viral infection	Lymphopenia, decreased T cells, depressed helper/suppressor ratio	None	None	None
Chronic infection	Usually none	Increased immunoglobulins	Increased components	Decreased chemotaxis
Multiple or recurrent viral infection	Decreased T cells and helper cells	Increased immunoglobulins, IgA, and antibodies to virus	Unknown	Unknown
MALIGNANT NEOPLASMS				
Acute leukemia	Decreased delayed hypersensitivity	Variable immunoglobulin levels	Unknown	None
Chronic leukemia	Decreased lymphocyte stimulation	Variable immunoglobulin levels	Unknown	None
Hodgkin's disease	Suppression of T cells and of delayed hypersensitivity	Increased or normal immunoglobulins; decreased antibody response to some antigens	Unknown	Frequent pneumococcal and *Haemophilus influenza* infections; decreased chemotaxis
Myeloma	Increased T-suppressor cells	Impaired antibody response; decreased immunoglobulins	Decreased components	None
Nonlymphoid cancer	Variable decrease in delayed hypersensitivity; suppression of T-cells; presence of immunosuppressive factors	Variable immunoglobulin levels	Decreased components with some tumors	None
TREATMENTS				
Anesthesia	Inhibited function	Unknown	Unknown	Decreased phagocytosis
Corticosteroids	Transient decrease	Transient decrease; decreased immunoglobulin synthesis (late)	None	Inhibited release of lysosomal enzymes; decreased phagocytosis of IgG-coated particles
Cyclosporine	No change in T-cell number; depressed allograft rejection reaction	Inhibition of T cell–dependent antibody response	Unknown	Unknown
Cytotoxic drugs (alkylating agents, antimetabolites)	Decreased numbers and function (variable); suppressed or enhanced response	Decreased numbers and function (variable); impaired primary antibody response	None	Decreased neutrophil and monocyte production
Phenytoin, penicillamine	Unknown	IgA deficiency, hypogammaglobulinemia	Unknown	Unknown
Radiation	Decreased T cell numbers and function (may be prolonged)	Impaired antibody production	Unknown	Decreased monocytes (transient)

Continued

Primary and Secondary Immunodeficiency

Mechanisms of selected secondary immunodeficiencies—*continued*

	CELL-MEDIATED IMMUNITY	HUMORAL IMMUNITY		NONSPECIFIC IMMUNITY
Cause	**Effect on T cells**	**Effect on B cells**	**Effect on complement**	**Effect on phagocytosis**
OTHER FACTORS				
Aging	Decreased delayed hypersensitivity; decreased mitogen response and T cells; abnormal T-suppressor cells	Increased IgG or IgA; increased B cells; decreased IgG response to some antigens	Unknown	Unknown
Development (newborn and premature infants)	Increased T-suppressor cells	Decreased IgM and IgA; impaired antibody-forming ability for various antigens	Decreased complement factors; abnormal chemotaxis	Decreased killing
Malnutrition	Decreased delayed hypersensitivity; decreased T cells; lymphopenia	None	Decreased CH_{50}	Abnormal bacterial killing

Self-Test

1. Acquired immunodeficiency syndrome (AIDS) is the result of infection with the human immunodeficiency virus (HIV) and is characterized by the presence of one or more of the following: chronic wasting syndrome, dementia, and a variety of secondary opportunistic infections and malignancies.
a. true **b.** false

2. Transmission of HIV may occur through:
a. exposure to infected blood **b.** sexual contact with a person infected with HIV **c.** gestation or birth, to an infant of an infected mother **d.** all of the above

3. A positive enzyme-linked immunosorbent assay or Western Blot assay indicates that:
a. the patient has AIDS **b.** the patient has ARC **c.** the patient has been exposed to HIV and therefore has antibodies to it **d.** the patient has been exposed to HIV and therefore has antigen to it

4. The drug most commonly administered to patients with *Pneumocystis carinii* pneumonia is:
a. dapsone **b.** trimetrexate **c.** pyrimethamine **d.** trimethoprim-sulfamethoxazole

5. Immune globulin therapy may be indicated for all of the following disorders except:
a. severe combined immunodeficiency disease **b.** selective IgA deficiency **c.** Wiskott-Aldrich syndrome **d.** agammaglobulinemia

6. Treatment of severe combined immunodeficiency disease may include:
a. histocompatible bone marrow transplant **b.** immune globulin therapy **c.** fetal thymus tissue transplant **d.** all of the above

Answers (page number shows where answer appears in text)
1. **a** (page 68) 2. **d** (page 69) 3. **c** (page 81) 4. **d** (page 85) 5. **b** (page 108) 6. **d** (page 112)

Transplant-related Immunologic Problems: Understanding Rejection Reactions

Nancy R. Noedel, who wrote this chapter, is heart transplant nurse coordinator and manager of the heart transplant program at St. Louis University Hospital. Ms. Noedel received her BSN from St. Louis University and is currently an MSN candidate in cardiopulmonary nursing.

Most transplant complications occur because the patient's immune system distinguishes the transplanted organ as foreign and attacks it. To understand this process, called transplant rejection, you'll need to understand the interplay of antigens on the transplanted tissue, the recipient's immune response, and such response-modifiers as immunosuppression. This chapter will help you gain this understanding. It will prepare you to assess, prevent, and treat transplant rejection, including graft-versus-host (GVH) disease.

This chapter also summarizes immunologic considerations for selected transplant procedures, such as kidney and bone marrow transplants. But before discussing transplant rejection, we'll review the different types of grafts and the genetic factors that determine donor and recipient compatibility.

Classifying grafts

Grafts—tissues or organs used for transplantation—are classified according to the genetic relationship between the donor and the recipient. They include:

- *Allograft.* Formerly known as a homograft, an allograft refers to a transplant between genetically nonidentical individuals. Nearly all the transplants we discuss will be allografts.
- *Autograft.* In this type of graft, the patient's own tissue is transplanted. Commonly performed autografts include skin grafts from healthy sites grafted onto burned areas and autologous bone marrow infusion in patients with leukemia, lymphoma, or other malignant diseases.
- *Syngraft.* Formerly known as an isograft, a syngraft refers to a graft exchanged between genetically identical donor and recipient, such as monozygotic twins.
- *Xenograft.* Formerly known as a heterograft, a xenograft refers to a transplant involving members of different species. Surgeons, for instance, have transplanted hearts and kidneys from animals, such as baboons, into humans.

The role of MHC

A chromosomal region, the major histocompatibility complex (MHC) contains genes that code for cell surface antigens that, in turn, determine the survival or rejection of a transplant. MHC genes also influence immune responses to infections and susceptibility to immunologically mediated diseases.

In humans, the MHC antigens are called human leukocyte antigens (HLA). The HLA antigens may be found on the short arm of chromosome 6, in seven recognized loci:

- HLA-A
- HLA-B
- HLA-C
- HLA-D
- HLA-DR (HLA-D related)
- HLA-DQ (formerly HLA-DC, HLA-MB, or HLA-DS)
- HLA-DP (formerly HLA-SB).

Each of these loci contains alleles—pairs of genes that embody specific inheritable characteristics and are located on the same

Transplant-related Immunologic Problems

chromosomal site. Researchers use a number to identify alleles at each locus. For example, HLA-A1 is the number 1 allele at the HLA-A locus.

The HLA system is highly polymorphic, with multiple alleles at each locus. For example, the HLA-A locus contains at least 23 distinct alleles and the HLA-B locus at least 47. Each allele determines a product. HLA-A, HLA-B, HLA-C, HLA-D, HLA-DR, HLA-DQ, and HLA-DP alleles are responsible for antigenic determinants carried by cell-surface molecules. (See *HLA loci*.)

A combination of alleles on a single chromosome is called a *haplotype*. Each HLA haplotype is usually inherited as a unit. Because offspring inherit one chromosome from each parent, they possess two haplotypes. Because all HLA genes are co-dominant, both haplotypes are expressed and each cell includes two complete sets of HLA antigens.

According to simple Mendelian inheritance, two siblings have a 25% chance of sharing both haplotypes (HLA-identical), a 50% chance of sharing one haplotype (HLA–semi-identical), and a 25% chance of sharing no haplotype (HLA-nonidentical). Only rarely will two unrelated individuals be HLA-identical. The immune system may regard any HLA configuration different from the recipient's own as an antigen. As a result, any transplanted tissue that doesn't share the patient's HLA configuration may provoke an immune response.

Classifying HLA. HLA antigens are classified into two major groups, based on structure and tissue distribution.

Continued on page 124

HLA loci

The following is a complete list of recognized human leukocyte antigen (HLA) loci and their respective alleles. A "w" by the allele number (for example, HLA-DRw1) indicates that scientists have located but not yet officially recognized that allele.

HLA-A	HLA-B		HLA-C	HLA-D	HLA-DR	HLA-DQ	HLA-DP
A1	Bw4	Bw47	Cw1	Dw1	DR1	DQw1	DPw1
A2	B5	Bw48	Cw2	Dw2	DR2	DQw2	DPw2
A3	Bw6	Bw49(21)	Cw3	Dw3	DR3	DQw3	DPw3
A9	B7	Bw50(21)	Cw4	Dw4	DR4		DPw4
A10	B8	B51(5)	Cw5	Dw5	DR5		Dpw5
A11	B12	Bw52(5)	Cw6	Dw6	DRw6		DPw6
Aw19	B13	Bw53	Cw7	Dw7	DR7		
A23(9)	B14	Bw54(w22)	Cw8	Dw8	DRw8		
A24(9)	B15	Bw55(w22)		Dw9	DRw9		
A25(10)	B16	Bw56(w22)		Dw10	DRw10		
A26(10)	B17	Bw57(17)		Dw11(w7)	DRw11(5)		
A28	B18	Bw58(17)		Dw12	DRw12(5)		
A29(w19)	B21	Bw59		Dw13	DRw13(w6)		
A30(w19)	Bw22	Bw60(40)		Dw14	DRw14(w6)		
A31(w19)	B27	Bw61(40)		Dw15	DRw52		
A32(w19)	B35	Bw62(15)		Dw16	DRw53		
Aw33(w19)	B37	Bw63(15)		Dw17(w7)			
Aw34(10)	B38(16)	Bw64(14)		Dw18(w6)			
Aw36	B39(16)	Bw65(14)		Dw19(w6)			
Aw43	B40	Bw67					
Aw66(10)	Bw41	Bw70					
Aw68(28)	Bw42	Bw71(w70)					
Aw69(28)	B44(12)	Bw72(w70)					
	B45(12)	Bw73					
	Bw46						

Transplant-related Immunologic Problems

MHC structure

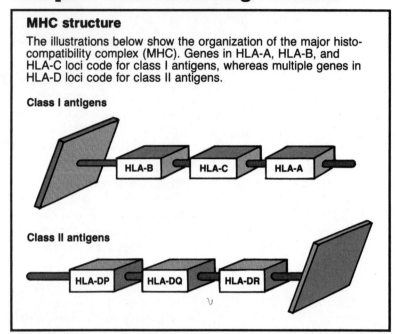

The illustrations below show the organization of the major histocompatibility complex (MHC). Genes in HLA-A, HLA-B, and HLA-C loci code for class I antigens, whereas multiple genes in HLA-D loci code for class II antigens.

Class I antigens

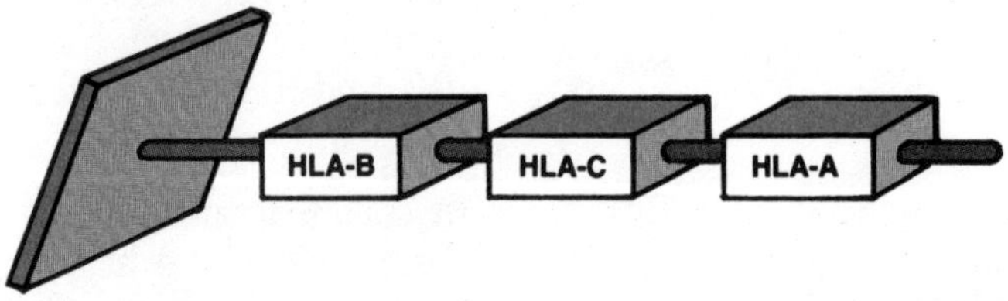

Class II antigens

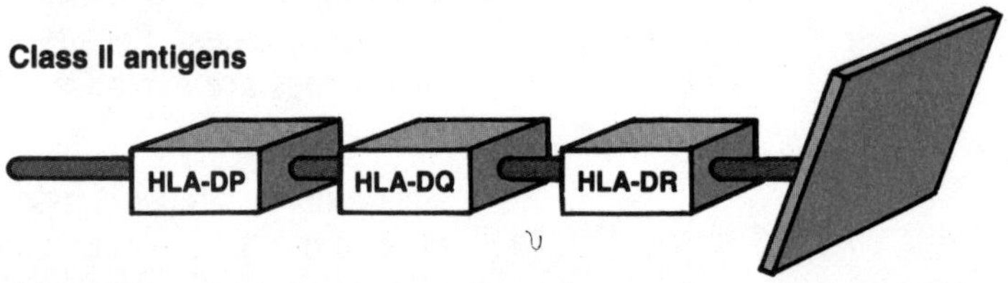

Continued

Class I antigens include the HLA-A, HLA-B, and HLA-C antigens. Widely distributed and found on every human nucleated cell except red blood cells (RBCs), class I antigens are the principal antigens recognized by the recipient during graft rejection.

Class II antigens, which include the HLA-D, HLA-DR, HLA-DQ, and HLA-DP antigens, appear mainly on the surfaces of immunocompetent cells, such as B cells, activated T cells, monocytes, and macrophages. Class II antigens facilitate interactions among immunologic cells. Strong evidence indicates that these antigens, either within the donor tissue itself or on leukocytes in the donor tissue, stimulate transplant rejection. They also initiate GVH disease, a frequent complication of bone marrow transplantation. (See *MHC structure*.)

In transplant rejection reactions, class I antigens serve as the main targets for killer (K) cells, while class II antigens carry the primary stimulating determinants for T-helper cells.

A third class of HLA antigens, class III antigens, contains genes that determine components C2 and C4 of the classic complement pathway and the properdin factor B of the alternate pathway.

Transplant rejection

The most frequent complication after transplantation, graft rejection occurs when the immune system recognizes the graft as nonself and responds to the foreign antigens. This recognition largely reflects the histocompatibility differences between donor and recipient.

Initially, the recipient's immune system recognizes antigens as foreign and conveys this information to the lymphoid centers. T-helper cells translate this information and a cell-mediated immune re-

Transplant-related Immunologic Problems

sponse takes place in the lymphoid tissues. This response leads to lymphocyte infiltration, lymphokine release, and eventual tissue necrosis. Other contributing mechanisms include:
- antibody-mediated immune responses
- the inflammatory response
- complement activation.

Transplant rejection may occur quickly or slowly, depending on the magnitude of antigenic differences between donor and recipient, and on any previous sensitization of the recipient to the donor's histocompatibility antigens. By altering the recipient's immune function, immunosuppressive treatment and illness may affect the onset of a rejection reaction.

Mechanisms of rejection
Transplant rejection can be classified as hyperacute, acute, or chronic, depending on the mechanism of rejection and the duration before signs of rejection appear. (For a summary of the three different mechanisms, see *Transplant rejection reactions,* page 126.)

Hyperacute rejection reactions. These develop within minutes (immediate) to a few days (accelerated) after transplantation.

An *immediate* hyperacute reaction occurs when the recipient has preformed antibodies against donor tissue antigens. These antibodies usually develop from previous blood transfusions, with leukocytes providing the sensitizing antigens. They may also result from pregnancy or an earlier transplant. In this type of reaction, antibodies cause complement activation and platelet aggregation, producing thrombosis in target tissues—mainly the vascular endothelium. This leads to acute ischemia, perhaps with hemorrhage, thrombosis, and loss of the graft.

An *accelerated* hyperacute reaction occurs when recipient lymphocytes and neutrophils infiltrate the graft. It's mediated by T cells rather than by antibodies. Treatment with antisera to T lymphocytes or thymocytes may prevent an accelerated reaction.

Acute rejection reactions. Acute rejection may begin by the end of the first week after transplantation. Immunosuppressive therapy, though, may delay onset for up to several weeks. Two types of acute rejection reactions may occur.

In a *cell-mediated* acute reaction, the graft develops interstitial edema, ischemia, and necrosis. High-dose corticosteroid therapy may reverse this reaction.

In an *antibody-mediated* acute reaction, fibrin, platelets, and polymorphonuclear cells adhere to graft cells and produce ischemia and necrosis. This reaction apparently results from antibodies produced by the recipient in response to donor antigens. Immunosuppressive therapy won't reverse this reaction.

Chronic rejection reactions. These develop over many months, leading to gradual loss of graft function. A chronic rejection reaction involves both cell-mediated and antibody-mediated responses. Histologic examination usually shows proliferation of the arterial intima and narrowing of the lumen, probably from chronic inflammation of the vascular endothelium. Fibrin and platelet ag-

Continued on page 126

Transplant-related Immunologic Problems

Transplant rejection reactions

Type of reaction	Duration after transplantation	Responsible immune mechanism
Hyperacute		
• immediate	Minutes	Preformed antibodies
• accelerated	1 to 5 days	T cells
Acute		
• cell-mediated	2 weeks or longer	Delayed hypersensitivity reaction
• antibody-mediated	1 week or longer	Antibodies
Chronic	Months to years	T cells and antibodies

Transplant rejection—*continued*

gregates form and incorporate immunoglobulins and complement. These aggregates eventually become covered with endothelium, resulting in decreased blood flow and ischemia to the graft. Immunosuppressive agents have little effect on this process. (For an example of immediate hyperacute, acute, and chronic rejection, see *Kidney transplant rejection*.)

Assessment

Detecting transplant rejection requires careful and accurate assessment. Unfortunately, however, assessing a patient for transplant rejection poses many difficulties. For instance:

- A patient may be asymptomatic or display only vague, nonspecific symptoms.
- Rejection may occur moments after transplantation, or it may occur months or even years later.
- Immunosuppressive drugs may alter assessment findings.

An accurate assessment hinges on a thorough health history, correlated with physical findings and laboratory test results.

History and physical examination. Signs and symptoms of rejection depend on the type of graft. (See *Signs and symptoms of transplant rejection,* page 129.) Commonly, the patient may have a low-grade fever and complain of malaise and fatigue. He also may experience other nonspecific complaints, such as anorexia, nausea, restlessness, or anxiety. Edema may cause him to gain weight.

Physical examination may reveal swelling, tenderness, and enlargement in the involved organ or site, especially in a patient who has undergone kidney, liver, or pancreas transplantation.

After transplantation, even if the patient appears asymptomatic, assess for signs of infection. Keep in mind that any change in a patient requires further investigation to rule out rejection. Inspect the skin surface—focusing on sites of injury, incision, or venipuncture—for signs of inflammation or delayed healing. Explore any complaints of altered bowel or bladder function, including changes in frequency, amount, color, consistency, and odor.

Diagnostic tests. Although graft survival often hinges on early detection of transplant rejection, no single test or combination of tests proves definitive. Tests reveal only nonspecific evidence, which

Continued on page 128

Transplant-related Immunologic Problems

Kidney transplant rejection

The illustrations below show the major mechanisms of immediate hyperacute, acute, and chronic kidney transplant rejection.

Immediate hyperacute rejection
In immediate hyperacute rejection, preexisting antibodies in the recipient's immune system enter the donor kidney and flood the capillaries of the renal cortex. This activates the complement and fibrinogen systems.

Complement activation triggers chemotaxis of polymorphonuclear cells, which infiltrate surrounding tissue and destroy endothelial cells.

Platelets adhere to denuded areas, which activates the coagulation system and leads to vascular occlusion.

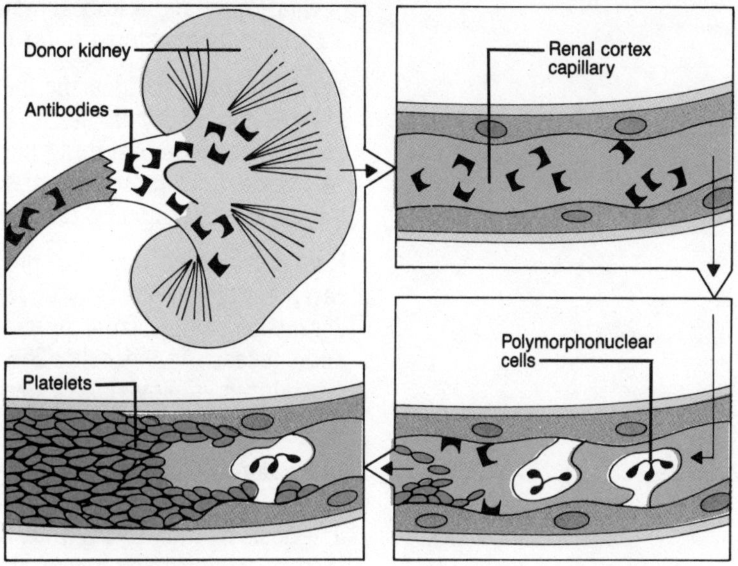

Acute rejection
In acute rejection, the recipient's lymph nodes process antigens from the donor kidney. Lymphocytes become sensitized, thus marking the beginning of cell-mediated and antibody-mediated responses.

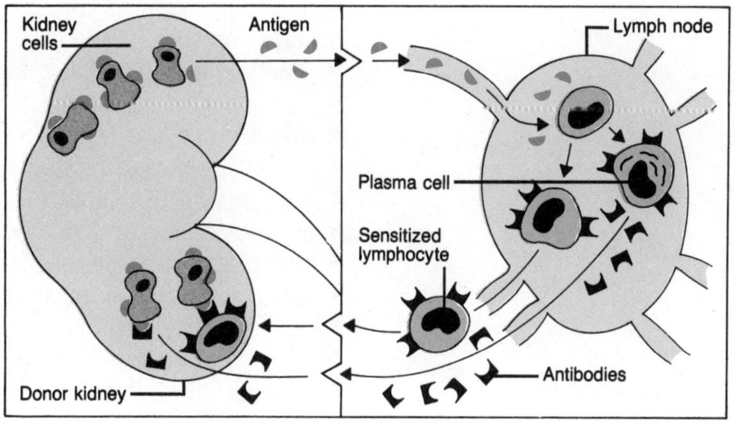

Chronic rejection
Antibodies and possibly sensitized lymphocytes penetrate the capillaries of the donor kidney, disrupting the endothelium and the glomerular basement membrane and causing protein leakage into the urinary space.

The body's repeated attempts to repair the damage result in endothelial proliferation, necrosis, collagen deposition, and, eventually, vascular occlusion.

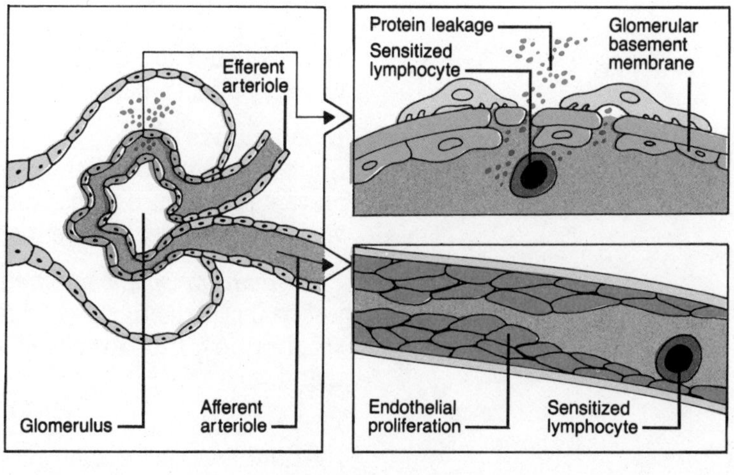

Transplant-related Immunologic Problems

Transplant rejection—*continued*

may easily be attributed to other causes, especially infection. Diagnosis often becomes a matter of exclusion and depends on careful evaluation of signs and symptoms along with results from specific organ function tests, standard laboratory studies, and tissue biopsy.

Tissue biopsy provides the most accurate, reliable diagnostic information, especially in heart, liver, and kidney transplants. Biopsy usually involves obtaining several tissue samples, preparing them on slides, and examining them under a microscope to determine the extent of lymphocytic infiltration and tissue damage.

Repeat biopsies may also prove beneficial. They can help identify early histologic changes characteristic of rejection, determine the degree of change from previous biopsies, and monitor the course and success of treatment. The frequency of biopsies and the specific procedures employed vary depending on the type of transplant, the hospital protocol, and the patient's history and health status.

Planning

Before determining your nursing care plan, develop the nursing diagnosis by identifying your patient's problem or potential problem, then relating it to its cause. Possible nursing diagnoses for a patient with transplant rejection include:

- body temperature, potential alteration in; related to transplant rejection process
- infection, potential for; related to immunosuppression
- tissue perfusion, potential alteration in; related to transplant rejection process
- knowledge deficit; related to inadequate health teaching
- noncompliance; related to long-term drug therapy
- activity intolerance; related to transplant rejection process
- fear; related to potential transplant rejection or loss
- anxiety; related to unexpected hospitalization
- skin integrity, impairment of; related to surgery
- comfort, alteration in (pain); related to surgery
- self-concept, disturbance in body image; related to transplantation.

The sample nursing care plan on page 130 shows expected outcomes, nursing interventions, and discharge planning for one nursing diagnosis listed above. However, you'll want to tailor each care plan to your patient's particular needs.

Interventions

Starting even before a transplant takes place, interventions aim to prevent rejection. If transplant rejection develops despite these preventive measures, interventions seek to treat the reaction.

Preventing transplant rejection. Measures to prevent transplant rejection include antigen matching, tissue typing, tests to detect prior sensitization, transfusions of whole blood, and immunosuppressive therapy.

Antigen matching, which involves matching the class I and class II HLA antigens (especially the HLA-B antigens) of donor and recip-

Continued on page 130

Transplant-related Immunologic Problems

Signs and symptoms of transplant rejection

To help ensure early detection of transplant rejection, be alert for the signs and symptoms listed below. Note that most transplant patients experience at least one rejection episode.

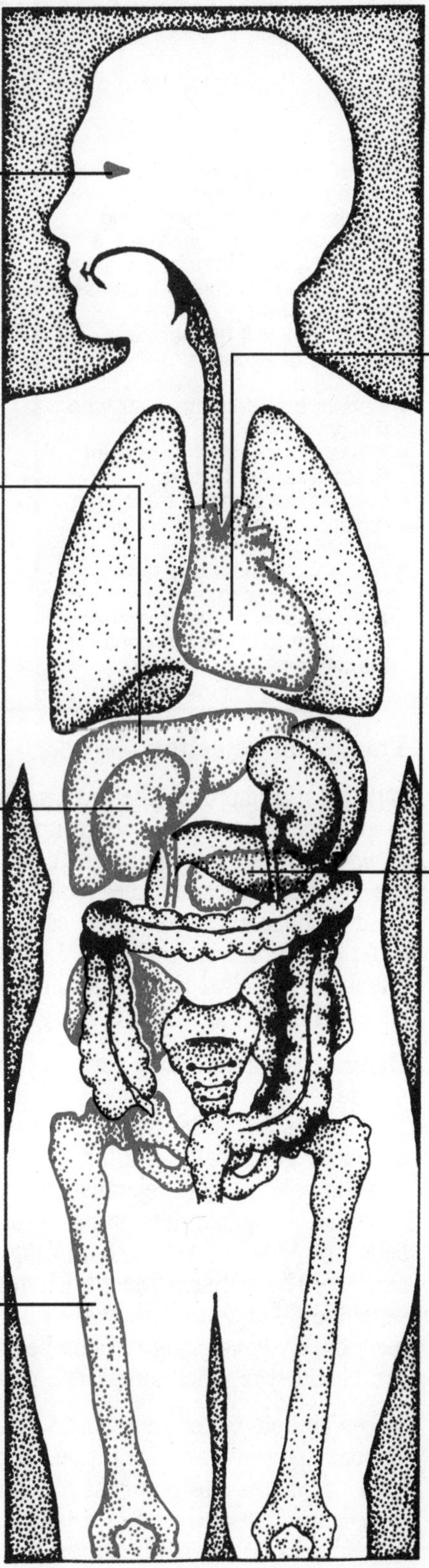

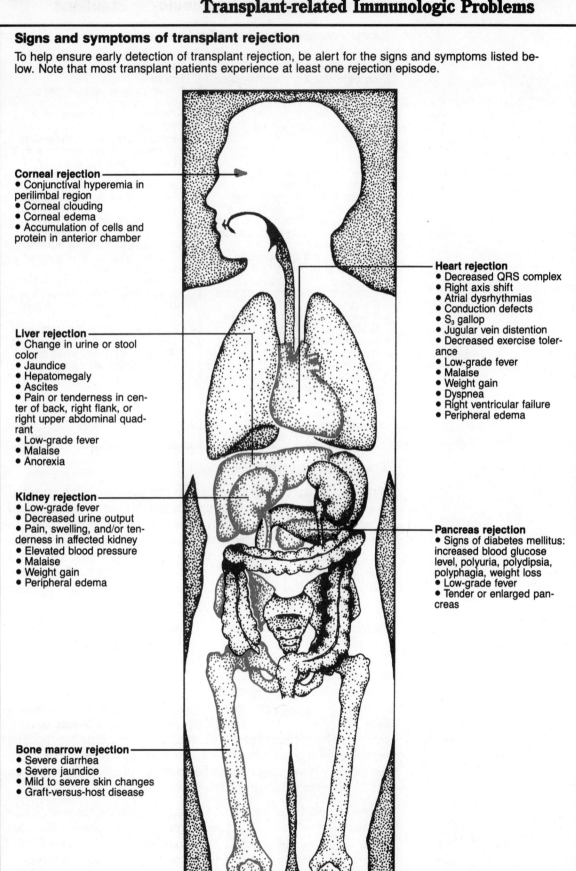

Corneal rejection
- Conjunctival hyperemia in perilimbal region
- Corneal clouding
- Corneal edema
- Accumulation of cells and protein in anterior chamber

Heart rejection
- Decreased QRS complex
- Right axis shift
- Atrial dysrhythmias
- Conduction defects
- S_3 gallop
- Jugular vein distention
- Decreased exercise tolerance
- Low-grade fever
- Malaise
- Weight gain
- Dyspnea
- Right ventricular failure
- Peripheral edema

Liver rejection
- Change in urine or stool color
- Jaundice
- Hepatomegaly
- Ascites
- Pain or tenderness in center of back, right flank, or right upper abdominal quadrant
- Low-grade fever
- Malaise
- Anorexia

Kidney rejection
- Low-grade fever
- Decreased urine output
- Pain, swelling, and/or tenderness in affected kidney
- Elevated blood pressure
- Malaise
- Weight gain
- Peripheral edema

Pancreas rejection
- Signs of diabetes mellitus: increased blood glucose level, polyuria, polydipsia, polyphagia, weight loss
- Low-grade fever
- Tender or enlarged pancreas

Bone marrow rejection
- Severe diarrhea
- Severe jaundice
- Mild to severe skin changes
- Graft-versus-host disease

Transplant-related Immunologic Problems

Sample nursing care plan: Transplant rejection

Nursing diagnosis	Expected outcomes
Body temperature, potential alteration in; related to transplant rejection process	The patient will: • maintain normal body temperature. • demonstrate adequate graft function. • state the signs and symptoms of transplant rejection for which he must remain alert.
Nursing interventions	**Discharge planning**
• Assess vital signs, including temperature, at least every 4 hours. Notify doctor of any changes—particularly increasing temperature. • Notify doctor if temperature reaches or exceeds 100.4° F. (38° C.). • Monitor for adequate graft functioning. • Assess for signs of transplant rejection and infection. • Discuss the signs of transplant rejection with the patient and his family. • Teach the patient and family members how to take a temperature reading properly, and advise them to notify the doctor if the patient's temperature reaches 100.4° F. or higher.	• Reinforce treatments and care plan. • Teach the patient and his family about the process of rejection, its diagnosis, and its treatment. • Explain what to do if signs of rejection develop. • Explain the importance of lifelong follow-up examinations to help ensure early detection of complications. • Arrange for follow-up care as needed. • Advise the patient when to seek medical attention.

Transplant rejection—*continued*

ient, greatly improves the graft's survival time. Also, it's essential to avoid certain ABO blood group incompatibilities. (See *ABO blood group antigens*.) The donor graft cannot contain antigens absent in the recipient because the recipient may have isohemagglutinins against those antigens. Other compatibility tests match ABO blood groups and Lewis antigens. Lewis antigen incompatibility may affect the survival time of renal allografts and may have additive effects if class I or class II antigens don't match.

Tissue typing refers to a series of tests that identify and compare a wide range of HLA antigens in the recipient and potential donors. The results are essential in evaluating histocompatibility because the more genetically similar the donor and recipient tissues, the less the possibility of rejection. Microtoxicity assays help detect the inherited antigenic determinants on cell surfaces. The recipient's cells are added to wells containing antisera and a source of complement. The antisera react with antigens on the lymphocytes and sensitize them so that they are killed when complement enters the reaction. By comparing the number of recipient cells killed, doctors can choose the most compatible donor.

Mixed leukocyte reactions offer additional information specifically for bone marrow transplantation. During the assay, blood leukocytes from the donor and recipient are mixed in vitro. The class II histocompatibility antigens of a potential donor stimulate deoxyribonucleic acid (DNA) synthesis in the recipient. The amount of DNA

Transplant-related Immunologic Problems

ABO blood group antigens

ABO blood group antigens form the basis of human blood group classifications. These antigens also appear in all body tissues except the brain and spinal cord. Like blood transfusion, organ transplantation depends on ABO compatibility:

- type O recipient receives a type O organ
- type A recipient receives a type A or O organ
- type B recipient receives a type B or O organ
- type AB recipient may receive a type AB, A, B, or O organ.

If a donor's erythrocytes carry foreign ABO antigens, a recipient may have isohemagglutinins against those antigens. Rapid graft rejection and injury to the vascular endothelium of the new organ may follow transplantation, probably because of antibodies directed against incompatible A or B antigens. (For more information on ABO grouping, see the NURSEREVIEW section on "Hematologic Problems.")

synthesis correlates with the genetic disparity between donor and recipient. Therefore, the donor who produces the smallest amount of DNA synthesis provides the best match for the recipient.

Tests to detect prior sensitization to donor antigens also help gauge the risk of transplant rejection. Once a patient is accepted for transplantation, expect him to undergo a lymphocyte antibody screen to reveal preformed antibodies in his blood. If preformed lymphocytotoxic antibodies appear in his serum, they could lead to an immediate hyperacute reaction and destruction of the graft after implantation. This makes the search for a suitable donor more difficult.

After finding a suitable donor, expect the donor to undergo a lymphocyte cross-match using the recipient's serum and the donor's T cells and B cells. If the cross-match reveals that the recipient's serum contains preformed antibodies against donor antigens, it indicates a high risk of hyperacute transplant rejection.

Whole blood transfusions administered to the recipient before transplantation seem to improve the prospects of graft survival in some organs. The reasons for this effect remain unclear.

Immunosuppressive drug therapy aims to decrease or eliminate the body's ability to reject the newly grafted tissue. While inducing tolerance to the graft, drug therapy also attempts to leave the immune system intact enough to protect against pathogens. However, the immunosuppressed patient faces an increased risk for serious—sometimes potentially fatal—infection from such opportunistic organisms as cytomegalovirus, fungi, mycobacteria, and protozoa. The high level of immunosuppression attained just after the procedure increases the patient's risk during the first few months of therapy. The therapy also increases the danger of developing such neoplastic disease as lymphoma.

Despite the potential drawbacks, however, immunosuppressive drug therapy remains the cornerstone of preventing and treating transplant rejection. Nearly all transplant recipients receive immunosuppressive drugs before and for some time after the procedure.

Usually, therapy involves some combination of drugs rather than a single agent. Commonly used drugs include antilymphocyte globulin, azathioprine, corticosteroids, cyclosporine, and muromonab-CD3. Other agents currently under investigation include anti–T cell monoclonal antibodies, cyclophosphamide, genetically engineered lymphoid-specific chalones, high-dose interferon, methotrexate, niridazole, oxisuran, procarbazine hydrochloride, and prostaglandin analogues. Dosages vary widely, depending on the type of transplant and the preference of the transplant team.

Several nondrug interventions, including radiation therapy and thoracic duct drainage, also show promise in providing pretransplant immunosuppression.

Antilymphocyte globulin, also known as antithymocyte globulin, lymphocyte immune globulin, or antisera, is an immunoglobulin produced from horse or rabbit antisera and frequently used to treat acute graft rejection. Injection of antilymphocyte globulin helps to

Continued on page 132

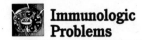

Transplant-related Immunologic Problems

Transplant rejection—*continued*

reduce the number of circulating lymphocytes. The drug provides adjunctive therapy to allograft recipients who can't tolerate corticosteroids or other drugs. Researchers are also investigating its use in treating autoimmune disorders. This drug impairs both T-cell and B-cell function and produces a reversible lymphocytopenia. Its major adverse effects include increased susceptibility to infection and, occasionally, allergic reactions (anaphylaxis and serum sickness).

Expect the doctor to order *azathioprine* postoperatively, usually in combination with corticosteroids and cyclosporine. When used in combination therapy, azathioprine helps to minimize the adverse effects of cyclosporine and may allow reduction of the cyclosporine dosage. In addition, combination therapy usually provides a greater degree of immunosuppression than drugs used alone.

Azathioprine affects nucleic acid synthesis in rapidly dividing cells, particularly lymphocytes, by interfering with purine synthesis. This reduces proliferation of white blood cells (WBCs) from the bone marrow. Because the drug is selective for T cell–mediated responses, it suppresses cell-mediated immunity but leaves antibody-mediated immunity relatively intact. Inhibiting effects on T-cell function help to ensure graft acceptance but also increase susceptibility to infection and cancer. Azathioprine can produce serious adverse effects, including bone marrow suppression (especially monocytopenia and neutropenia), macrocytic anemia, hepatitis, and pancreatitis.

Expect to administer *corticosteroids* (particularly prednisone and methylprednisolone) with cyclosporine to help prevent transplant rejection. Corticosteroids may also treat a rejection reaction once it occurs. Their effect on the immune system remains somewhat unclear, but corticosteroids influence circulation of WBCs, thereby inducing eosinopenia, lymphopenia, monocytopenia, and neutrophilia. They also impair macrophage and granulocyte mediator release, and alter the cell-mediated immune response. In high doses, corticosteroids probably stimulate cytokine release, affecting T-cell and macrophage collaboration.

Because corticosteroids exert an anti-inflammatory influence, their use can result in delayed wound healing and increased susceptibility to infection. Other potential adverse effects include hyperglycemia, hypertension, fluid retention, psychosis, characteristic cushingoid signs (hirsutism, moon face, buffalo hump, purple striae), and gastric ulcers. Long-term use can lead to osteoporosis, aseptic necrosis of weight-bearing joints, cataracts, and inhibited growth in children.

Cyclosporine, often given in combination with corticosteroids and other immunosuppressants, helps prevent acute rejection in various organ transplants and GVH disease in bone marrow transplants. By inhibiting production and release of interleukin-2, cyclosporine selectively inhibits T-cell proliferation, cytotoxicity, and lymphokine production, thus blocking the cell-mediated immune response in graft rejection.

Cyclosporine acts quickly. Once the immune response begins, however, cyclosporine appears ineffective in halting or reversing the

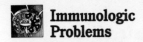

Transplant-related Immunologic Problems

rejection process. In addition, cyclosporine appears able to inhibit lymphocytes only after they have been exposed to a stimulating antigen. Administering the drug before transplantation doesn't improve the chances of allograft survival.

Dosage is highly individualized and may be regulated by measuring serum levels. Patients may receive a loading dose 12 hours before transplantation. Common adverse effects include nephrotoxicity, hepatotoxicity, central nervous system toxicity, and hypertension. These effects can often be minimized by reducing the drug dosage. Cyclosporine allows reduction of the corticosteroid dosage.

Muromonab-CD3, a monoclonal antibody, helps prevent kidney transplant rejection. Researchers are investigating its use in liver, heart, and pancreas transplants. This drug blocks T-cell effector functions involved in allograft rejection by recognizing and binding with the CD3 complex chain on T-cell antigen receptors. This decreases expression of the T-cell antigen receptor, thereby lessening the ability of T cells to recognize antigen. Its adverse effects include a flu-like syndrome with fever, headache, and gastric upset, which frequently appears at the start of therapy.

Treating transplant rejection. Once initiated, the immune response is difficult to suppress. Treatment focuses on minimizing the intensity of the immunologic attack on the transplanted tissue. Several drugs can improve graft survival during episodes of acute rejection reactions, although they haven't proven effective in treating hyperacute or chronic rejection reactions.

Corticosteroids can help control 60% to 75% of acute transplant rejection reactions, and they act quickly to help control the rejection process. Patients usually receive methylprednisolone sodium succinate I.V. until evidence indicates reversal of the rejection process. The doctor may order *antilymphocyte globulin* in conjunction with corticosteroid therapy; this combination has proven especially effective in treating rejection reactions that involve cell-mediated immune responses.

Muromonab-CD3 also may effectively reverse an acute rejection reaction, particularly in a kidney transplant. It produces marked lymphopenia, especially of T cells, and usually improves graft function in 2 to 7 days. *Cyclosporine* also may reverse acute rejection.

Currently, no effective treatment exists for chronic rejection reactions except retransplantation. In certain transplants, antiplatelet therapy may help decrease platelet aggregation and impede development of atherosclerosis in the graft.

Maintenance therapy. Most allograft recipients receive immunosuppressive therapy for as long as the graft continues to function. Doctors most commonly order prednisone on a daily or every-other-day schedule in combination with azathioprine. Patients have also benefited from immunosuppressive therapy with cyclosporine.

Evaluation

Base your evaluation on the expected outcomes listed on the nursing care plan. To determine if the patient has improved, ask yourself the following questions:

- Is the patient's body temperature within normal range?

Continued on page 134

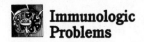

Transplant-related Immunologic Problems

Transplant rejection—*continued*

- Does the patient have adequate graft function?
- Does he exhibit any signs of transplant rejection?
- Can the patient identify and discuss the signs of transplant rejection?
- Does he know when to seek medical care for such signs?
- Does he understand important infection-prevention measures?
- Does he know what to do if he develops a fever?

The answers to these questions will help you evaluate your patient's status and the effectiveness of his care. Keep in mind that these questions stem from the sample nursing care plan on page 130. Your questions may differ.

GVH disease

GVH disease may occur when an immunologically impaired recipient receives a graft from an immunocompetent donor. If donor and recipient cells are not histocompatible, the foreign cells may launch an attack against the host cells, which are unable to reject them. The disease may occur even if extensive pre-transplant testing of both donor and recipient fails to uncover antigenic disparities.

This process begins when graft cells become sensitized to the recipient's class II antigens. The exact mechanism by which this occurs remains unclear, although biopsy of active GVH lesions usually reveals infiltration by mononuclear cells, eosinophils, and phagocytic and histiocytic cells.

GVH disease usually develops after a patient with impaired immune function—from congenital immunodeficiency, radiation treatments, or immunosuppressive drugs—receives a bone marrow transplant. However, it may also result from the transfusion of any blood product containing viable lymphocytes. This means that patients may develop GVH disease during the transfusion of whole blood or transplantation of fetal thymus, liver, or bone marrow. The risk of GVH disease transmission also exists during maternal-fetal blood transfusions and intrauterine transfusions.

GVH disease usually affects the skin, liver, GI tract, and, in some cases, the bone marrow. Onset may occur from 7 to 20 days following infusion of the viable lymphocytes. It proves fatal in about one third of affected patients.

Assessment. Signs of acute GVH disease include skin rash, severe diarrhea, and jaundice. Skin rash usually develops 10 to 28 days after transplantation. It typically begins as a diffuse erythematous macular rash on the palms, soles, and scalp and may spread to the trunk and possibly the extremities. In severe GVH disease, the rash can become desquamative. Abdominal cramps and, in severe cases, GI bleeding may accompany watery diarrhea. Jaundice results from the hyperbilirubinemia caused by inflammation of the small bile ducts, possibly accompanied by elevated serum alkaline phosphatase, alanine aminotransferase, and aspartate aminotransferase levels. Skin, intestine, and liver biopsies reveal immunocompetent T cells.

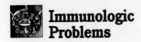

Transplant-related Immunologic Problems

Scientists at the University of Washington have developed a standard staging and grading system for acute GVH disease. (See *Stages of acute GVH disease*.)

Intervention. Because patients may die from GVH disease, initial interventions must focus on prevention. Most patients receive immunosuppressive drug therapy with methotrexate, cyclosporine, or cyclophosphamide for the first 3 to 12 months after transplantation. Other strategies to decrease the incidence of GVH disease involve attempting to deplete donor marrow of T cells. One method is to incubate donor bone marrow in vitro with anti–T cell monoclonal antibodies plus complement or similar antibodies coupled with toxins. Another technique for depleting marrow of T cells employs soybean lectin agglutination and sheep RBC rosette formation. Doctors may also isolate the recipient in a room with laminar air flow. For some reason, however, this measure has proven effective only in patients with aplastic anemia.

In treating established GVH disease, doctors have had limited success with infusions of antilymphocyte globulin, prednisone, cyclosporine, and in vivo monoclonal antibodies. Research on preventing and treating GVH disease has yielded two promising new experimental techniques: culturing of human bone marrow cells and use of thalidomide.

Culturing of bone marrow cells. Researchers are investigating the potential for autogenic transplants of cultured bone marrow cells. Growing cultures of hematopoietic stem cells in the presence of

Continued on page 136

Stages of acute GVH disease

Developed at the University of Washington, this system grades different stages of acute graft-versus-host (GVH) disease based on type and extent of rash, the degree of hyperbilirubinemia, and amount of diarrhea or other GI symptoms.

Stage	Skin	Bilirubin level*	GI symptoms
I	Maculopapular rash covering 25% or less of body surface	2 to 3 mg/dl (34 to 51 μmole/liter)	>0.5 liter of diarrhea/day
II	Maculopapular rash covering 25% to 50% of body surface	3 to 6 mg/dl (51 to 103 μmole/liter)	>1 liter of diarrhea/day
III	Generalized erythroderma	6 to 15 mg/dl (103 to 257 μmole/liter)	>1.5 liters of diarrhea/day
IV	Generalized erythroderma with bullous formation and desquamation	>15 mg/dl (>257 μmole/liter)	Severe abdominal pain, with or without ileus

**Note:* Normal bilirubin range is 0.1 to 1.0 mg/dl (2 to 18 μmole/liter).

Transplant-related Immunologic Problems

GVH disease—*continued*

marrow-derived stromal cells promotes growth of normal stem cells but suppresses production of leukemic cells. The marrow can then be reinfused to the patient, thereby reducing the risk of GVH disease.

Thalidomide. This drug binds to lymphocytes at the same intracellular receptors as cyclosporine and helps the immune system recognize both host and donor tissues as "self," thus reducing the risk of GVH disease. Although thalidomide causes teratogenic effects, chemotherapy and total body irradiation render transplant patients sterile. Adverse effects reportedly are limited to fatigue and possibly peripheral neuropathy.

Preventive measures. Patients suspected of having cellular immunodeficiency should receive only blood and blood products (including whole blood, packed RBCs, leukocyte-poor RBCs, and fresh plasma) that have been irradiated with 3,000 to 6,000 roentgens. Such irradiation destroys viable lymphocytes.

Chronic GVH disease. If acute GVH disease occurs 30 to 70 days after transplantation, it nearly always indicates the development of chronic GVH disease. An autoimmune disease, chronic GVH produces severe immunodeficiency leading to recurrent and life-threatening infections. Its signs and symptoms resemble collagen-vascular or autoimmune disorders. Older patients and those who have suffered previous acute GVH disease face the greatest risk of chronic GVH disease. Treatment with prednisone, alone or in combination with azathioprine, reverses many effects of chronic GVH disease in 50% to 75% of patients. Researchers are also investigating the use of a monoclonal antibody, XomaZyme-H65, to treat chronic GVH disease.

Besides the general principles presented in this chapter, you'll need to know specific pre-transplant and post-transplant care measures based on the type of transplant involved. On the following pages, a chart of selected organ and tissue transplants presents this information.

Transplant-related Immunologic Problems

Selected organ and tissue transplants

The following chart focuses on immunologic considerations for selected organ and tissue transplants. (For more information on individual procedures, see the appropriate NURSEREVIEW sections.)

BONE MARROW TRANSPLANT

Purpose

A bone marrow transplant may restore immunologic and hematologic function in patients with severe combined immunodeficiency disorder (SCID), aplastic anemia, or various leukemias, including acute and chronic myelogenous leukemia.

Pre-transplant measures

- Donor and recipient will undergo antigen matching, tissue typing, and leukocyte cross-matching.
- Immunosuppressive therapy usually includes cyclophosphamide for 2 to 4 days. Recipients may also receive total body irradiation in fractions over 3 to 5 days to avoid pulmonary and ocular toxicity. Total dose equals 7.5 to 15 Gy.
- Don't expect to provide immunosuppressive therapy if donor and recipient are HLA-matched or if the recipient has SCID.
- Partially matched recipients usually receive cyclophosphamide and busulfan rather than radiation therapy.
- Omitting radiation therapy reduces complications as well as toxicity but increases the risk of rejection.
- When parents of HLA–semi-identical children serve as donors, the surgical team may remove T cells from donor marrow by lectin agglutination or monoclonal antibody and complement lysis.
- If donor and recipient aren't ABO-compatible, either the recipient must undergo plasmapheresis to remove anti-A or anti-B antibodies or the surgeon must remove red blood cells (RBCs) from the marrow cells in vitro.

Procedure

With the donor under general or epidural anesthesia, the surgeon performs multiple aspirations of bone marrow of 5 ml each, yielding a total of about 10 ml/kg of the recipient's weight. The surgeon draws donor marrow through heparinized needles and places it into heparinized, buffered culture medium. He then gently filters this mixture through fine stainless steel mesh screens to produce a single cell suspension. A nucleated cell count helps to ensure the adequacy of withdrawn marrow. To perform the transplant, the surgeon infuses bone marrow cells intravenously together with RBCs.

Post-transplant care

- Expect to administer broad-spectrum antibacterial antibiotics (penicillins, cephalosporins, aminoglycosides) as well as acyclovir and amphotericin B. Continue antibiotics until absolute neutrophil counts pass 500/μl.
- To prevent severe spontaneous hemorrhage, expect to administer platelet transfusions. Maintain platelet count above 15,000/μl.
- To prevent infection, employ air filtration to remove airborne fungi and observe simple precautions such as hand-washing.
- As ordered, maintain isolation in a laminar airflow room for a patient with aplastic anemia.
- Before administering any blood product, be sure it has been irradiated. This will help to prevent graft-versus-host (GVH) disease caused by viable lymphocytes in the transformed cellular components or plasma.
- Monitor the patient for signs of infection, bleeding disorders, and GVH disease. Administer immunosuppressive therapy, as ordered.
- During the next 2 to 4 weeks, monitor the patient for signs of engraftment. Watch for a rising white blood cell (WBC) count, relative monocytosis, and the appearance of circulating neutrophils. Also at this time, bone marrow samples show increasing cellularity, and platelet and reticulocyte counts begin to rise.

Special considerations

- Until recently, most donors for bone marrow transplants have been identical twins or HLA-identical siblings. Expect only about one fourth of all patients to have an HLA-identical donor. Doctors are beginning to have more success with partially matched family members and phenotypically matched unrelated donors.
- Patients under age 30 who receive bone marrow transplant soon after diagnosis achieve the most favorable results. Diagnostic tests show that the Philadelphia chromosome may remain absent for as long as 5 years after the procedure. Transplants for patients with acute lymphoblastic leukemia haven't been as successful.
- The donor usually regenerates bone marrow in 8 weeks and suffers no immunologic or hematologic harm. Only about 20% of the donor's total marrow is harvested before the procedure.

BONE TRANSPLANT

Purpose

Bone transplant promotes healing of ununited fractures, restores skeletal structure integrity, or aids in cosmetic repair.

Pre-transplant measures

- An autograft is the preferred method of bone transplantation. But when autograft sources are insufficient, the surgeon may use allogeneic bone in combination with an autograft. To procure bone for implantation, the surgeon must remove it aseptically or sterilize it with ethylene oxide or gamma radiation.
- To reduce immunogenicity, expect to freeze all bone tissue except fresh autografts.

Procedure

The surgeon grafts bone in place of a removed bone or bony defect.

Post-transplant care

- Expect to provide temporary systemic immunosuppression for the next 2 to 3 months, typically with corticosteroids, cyclosporine, azathioprine, or cyclophosphamide. Immunosuppression is temporary because major histocompatibility complex (MHC) antigens remain on bone cells for a short time after transplantation.
- After the graft, the bone may:
  —become viable, acquiring the mechanical, cosmetic, and biologic characteristics of adjacent bone
  —partially or completely resorb without satisfactory new bone formation, leaving disfigurement or instability
  —become sequestrated and encapsulated. If so, the host will treat it as a foreign body.
- Assess for proper bone graft healing. Proper healing follows a well-defined pattern. For the first two weeks, you'll see inflammation, accompanied by the development of fibrous granulation tissue and infiltration with vascular buds. Osteoclast activity and osteocyte autolysis also occur. The graft will strengthen as mesenchymal cells differentiate into osteoblasts that deposit osteoid over devitalized trabeculae. Cortical bone grafts may take 1 to 2 years to reach full strength, cancellous bone grafts about half that time.
- Monitor for signs of graft rejection. A low-grade, slow, inflammatory response (characterized by pannus reaction and an increase in synovial fluid, WBC counts, and antibody response) indicates an immune response. Rejection of allogeneic bone delays processes that strengthen the graft: revascularization, resorption, and appositional bone formation.

Continued

Transplant-related Immunologic Problems

Selected organ and tissue transplants —*continued*

BONE TRANSPLANT—*continued*

Special considerations

• Remember that bone consists of cells, collagen, ground substance, and inorganic materials. Except for inorganic materials, all components are potentially immunogenic. MHC antigens are found on osteogenic, chondrogenic, fibrous, neuronal, fatty, hematopoietic, and mesenchymal cells, all of which are involved in bone allografts. The presence of cell-rich bone marrow also enhances immunogenicity.
• Keep in mind that fresh allogeneic bone may sensitize the host and induce production of circulating antibodies. Nevertheless, researchers believe that cellular immunity is usually more significant in transplant rejection than antibody immunity. Cartilage provides only partial protection against destruction by antibody-mediated and cell-mediated mechanisms.

HEART TRANSPLANT

Purpose

This transplant attempts to restore function in patients with end-stage cardiac disease who fail to respond to other treatments. Most often, these patients suffer from coronary artery disease, cardiomyopathy, rheumatic heart disease, congenital heart disease, or benign cardiac tumors.

Pre-transplant measures

• Donors and recipients undergo HLA-typing. The recipient will undergo a careful cross-match test to screen for preformed HLA antibodies. The number of eligible recipients is usually quite low.
• The donor heart will usually be taken from an individual under 40 years of age, with established neurologic death, no history of cardiac disease, and no abnormalities on chest X-rays or an EKG.
• Preserving optimal cardiac function and perfusion of the donor heart requires hydration and use of vasopressors and inotropic agents.
• Upon removing the donor heart, the surgical team will flush the coronary circulation with mixed-electrolyte solution and preserve the heart on ice. The surgeon must implant the heart within 4 hours after removal from donor.

Procedure

After placing the patient on cardiopulmonary bypass, the surgeon excises the diseased heart. He then implants the donor heart.

Post-transplant care

• As ordered, provide immunosuppressive therapy with corticosteroids, cyclosporine, or antilymphocyte globulin.
• The doctor may perform an endomyocardial biopsy to diagnose allograft rejection by placing a transvenous catheter in a right jugular vein. The presence of mononuclear cell infiltrates, such as lymphocytes, lymphoblasts, and monocytes, indicates rejection. Necrosis of myocardial fibers and edema indicate tissue damage. EKG may show decreased voltage and dysrhythmias. Signs of congestive heart failure may appear.
• Expect to treat rejection with antilymphocyte globulin and increasing levels of corticosteroids.
• Atherosclerotic changes in coronary vessels indicate chronic rejection.

Special considerations

• Combined heart-lung transplantation, with a higher success rate than lung transplant alone, has become the procedure of choice for patients with intractable pulmonary hypertension. The procedure involves anastomosis of the trachea, right atrium, and aorta. Immunosuppressive therapy may include cyclosporine, azathioprine, and antilymphocyte globulin, with corticosteroids added once tracheal healing has occurred.
• Endomyocardial biopsy detects combined heart-lung rejection, since heart rejection usually occurs simultaneously with lung rejection. Chest X-rays can indirectly diagnose lung rejection.

KIDNEY TRANSPLANT

Purpose

This transplant restores kidney function in patients with end-stage renal disease.

Pre-transplant measures

• Recipients and donors will undergo ABO red cell testing. If tests show ABO incompatibility, the doctor will not perform the transplant. ABO antigens are present on the vascular endothelium of the graft as well as on RBCs.
• Recipients and donors will undergo HLA-testing. Testing most likely will include the cross-match to detect preformed antibodies to donor HLA antigens.
• Expect to perform random blood transfusions in patients awaiting cadaveric transplantation. This may eliminate immunologic responders that demonstrate cytotoxic antibodies and lead to development of T-suppressor cells and blocking or anti-idiotypic antibodies.
• Expect to perform donor-specific transfusions (DSTs) in patients awaiting transplants from related donors. The DSTs will lead to induction of T-suppressor cells, development of blocking or anti-idiotypic antibodies, and clonal deletion.

Procedure

The surgical team implants the kidney by an iliac incision, placing the graft in the retroperitoneal position against the psoas muscle. Most likely the surgical team will anastomose the renal artery to the internal or external iliac artery and anastomose the renal vein to the external iliac vein.

Post-transplant care

• Carefully monitor renal function by evaluating serum electrolytes, blood urea nitrogen, and serum creatinine levels.
• To optimize renal perfusion and function, maintain hemodynamic status with fluid therapy.
• Expect to provide immunosuppressive therapy tailored to the patient's needs. Usually, the patient receives corticosteroids, possibly supplemented by cyclosporine, azathioprine, antilymphocyte globulin, or muromonab-CD3.
• The recipient may require plasmapheresis to remove lymphocytes and immunoglobulin.

Special considerations

• Because cadaveric kidneys usually have some degree of acute tubular necrosis, up to 50% of recipients of these kidneys may require dialysis.

LIVER TRANSPLANT

Purpose

This transplant attempts to restore liver function in patients with:
• hepatitis B antigen-negative postnecrotic cirrhosis
• chronic active hepatitis
• primary hepatocellular tumor
• congenital or developmental anomalies of the bile duct (in infants and children)

Continued

Transplant-related Immunologic Problems

Selected organ and tissue transplants—*continued*

LIVER TRANSPLANT—*continued*

• inborn errors of metabolism, such as tyrosinemia and Wilson's disease (in children).

Pre-transplant measures
• Recipients and donors undergo ABO typing, but not HLA matching. Doctors also look at organ size when evaluating the suitability of the transplant.

Procedure
Typically, the patient undergoes an orthotopic transplant. In this procedure, the surgeon removes the host liver and places a cadaver allograft in the right upper quadrant. In a heterotopic transplant, the surgeon places a liver at an ectopic site.

In an orthotopic transplant, the surgical team will retrieve the donor liver as the hepatectomy begins, flush it with cold solutions, and place it in hypothermic storage to be used within the next 6 to 10 hours.

The surgeon implants the donor liver by anastomosing the hepatic inferior vena cava to the recipient's vena cava and anastomosing the donor portal vein to the recipient's portal vein. He will then sew the infrahepatic vena cava to the donor inferior vena cava and the donor celiac artery to the common hepatic artery. Usually the bile duct is sewn to the recipient's common bile duct, though it may be connected to a Roux-en-Y loop of jejunum.

Post-transplant care
• Monitor for signs and symptoms of graft rejection, including fever, upper abdominal pain, decreased appetite, ascites, and hepatomegaly. Laboratory studies may show elevated levels of serum bilirubin, alkaline phosphatase, and transaminase as well as prolonged prothrombin time. Liver scans will usually show poor concentrations of radionuclides. The doctor may order a liver biopsy to help diagnose rejection.
• Expect to treat rejection with cyclosporine, along with corticosteroids and azathioprine.

Special considerations
• Both the patient's status and the donor organ supply will influence the doctor's decision whether to perform a liver transplant. Before transplant, the patient should show no signs of severe systemic complications from liver disease.

PANCREAS TRANSPLANT

Purpose
A pancreas transplant provides biologically responsive insulin-producing tissue in patients with insulin-dependent diabetes mellitus. The procedure prevents vascular changes associated with diabetes and helps to improve the patient's quality of life.

Pre-transplant measures
• Recipients and donors undergo typing and matching for ABO blood groups and HLA.
• The surgical team removes the pancreas from the donor and preserves it in cold storage up to 6 hours before the procedure.

Procedure
The surgeon implants either a whole pancreas with a small button of donor duodenum or a distal segment of the pancreas. Dispersed islets of Langerhans may also be transplanted.

For transplants from living related donors, the surgeon will use only segmental grafts. In this procedure, the surgeon removes about half of the pancreas body and tail and connects the vessels with the iliac vessels of the recipient. Alternatively, the surgeon may connect the celiac and portal vessels of the donor to the splenic vessels of the recipient. This will assure passage of venous effluent to the portal circulation.

Post-transplant care
• Monitor for signs of graft rejection. During rejection, expect to see loss of control over blood glucose levels. Unfortunately, you may easily attribute changes in blood glucose levels to other factors. Vasculitis, with parenchymal fibrosis and inflammatory cell infiltrates, provides a more definitive sign of rejection.
• Expect to treat rejection with corticosteroids, antilymphocyte globulin, or both.

Special considerations
• Unlike liver transplant, which may save a patient's life, pancreas transplant serves as a life-enhancing procedure, especially when performed before severe secondary diabetic complications develop. Otherwise, the risk of long-term immunosuppressive therapy may outweigh the risk of developing systemic complications of diabetes.

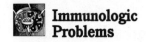

Tumor-related Immunologic Problems: Causes, Diagnosis, and Treatment

Joyce P. Griffin, who wrote this chapter, is an assistant professor of nursing at the University of Hawaii. Dr. Griffin received her BSN from the Herbert Lehman College of the City University of New York, her MSN from the Hunter College of the City University of New York, and her PhD from New York University.

This chapter reviews the antigenic properties of tumor cells, the immune response to tumor cells, and how the immune response aids tumor diagnosis and treatment. It also reviews how the immune system can be prompted to act against tumor cells.

The immune system and tumor growth

The immune system provides protection against malignant tumor growth—a formidable task considering that tumor cells have many similarities to normal cells. We'll first review the processes that render these cells different from normal ones. (See *Tumor cell traits*.)

Normal cells possess a variable capacity to proliferate. Tightly coordinated within a normal organ or tissue, cell loss roughly parallels new cell development. In disorders that stimulate cell proliferation, new cells may temporarily outnumber those needed for cell replacement; this polyclonal expansion causes organ or tissue hypertrophy. However, once this stimulus for cell growth is removed, cell proliferation subsides and hypertrophy reverses.

In contrast, tumor cells initially develop as normal cells but undergo a transformation, causing them to proliferate independently and uncontrollably.

Cell transformation

How do normal cells become malignant tumor cells? Some are transformed spontaneously by random mutations or genetic rearrangements; others are transformed by chemical, physical, or viral carcinogens. Just how this transformation occurs may have a bearing on the immune system's ability to recognize and control tumor growth. Oncogenic viruses, for instance, are most apt to activate the immune system. That's because cells transformed by viral genes usually express new virus-associated antigens that the immune system can recognize.

Oncogenic viruses can be divided into two types: deoxyribonucleic acid (DNA) and ribonucleic acid (RNA). Potentially oncogenic DNA viruses include papovaviruses, herpesviruses, and adenoviruses. Typically, infection with these viruses doesn't cause cancer. Furthermore, researchers haven't isolated oncogenic DNA viruses from human tumors. However, researchers do point to a link between a few viral infections and specific cancers. The implicated viruses include:

- herpes simplex virus (HSV) type 2, linked with cervical carcinoma
- Epstein-Barr virus (EBV), linked with Burkitt's lymphoma and nasopharyngeal carcinoma
- hepatitis B virus (HBV), linked with primary liver cancers.

Unlike DNA viruses, RNA viruses have a proven oncogenic role. These viruses contain genes for reverse transcriptase, which allows viral RNA to act as a template, transcribing a single-stranded DNA copy and then converting it into double-stranded DNA. This double strand can be inserted into the host tissue's genome. Because this process follows the opposite pattern of normal DNA-to-RNA transcription, these RNA viruses are called *retroviruses*.

Tumor cell traits

Tumor cells:

- are monoclonal in origin (However, as tumor mass increases, studies may detect genotypic and phenotypic heterogeneity.)
- fail to respond to the regulatory signals controlling normal growth and tissue repair
- grow without external stimulation
- invade normal tissues
- metastasize to distant organs via the lymphatic and circulatory systems
- appear different than normal cells from the same tissue.

Tumor-related Immunologic Problems

Oncogene-linked disorders

Oncogenes are viral genes with the potential to transform normal cells into neoplastic ones. Oncogenes found in RNA-containing retroviruses cause many malignancies. Although these viral genes are not specific to particular cancers, they tend to appear in certain malignancies. The following list includes the oncogenes identified so far and the disorders with which they're linked.

B lym-1	lymphoma
HER-2/neu	breast cancer
H-ras	carcinoma sarcoma
K-ras	leukemia lymphoma
met	osteosarcoma
myc	carcinoma sarcoma leukemia
N-myc	neuroblastoma
sis	simian sarcoma
src	chronic myelogenous leukemia lymphosarcoma

Retroviruses cause many naturally occurring cancers. For instance, human T-leukemia virus causes certain T-cell leukemias and lymphomas. Another retrovirus, human B-lymphotropic virus, is linked with lymphoid malignancies. Because many retroviruses spread readily from infected to normal cells, resistance to tumor growth depends partly on the immune response to the new virus-associated antigens.

Retroviruses can transform normal cells into tumor cells either rapidly or slowly. Rapidly transforming viruses contain oncogenes that alter cells directly. (See *Oncogene-linked disorders*.) Slowly transforming viruses lack oncogenes and must prompt host genes to induce the transformation. In either case, the resulting tumors are likely to express new surface antigens that the immune system can recognize.

Tumor antigens

Expressed by tumor cells, these antigens induce a cell- or antibody-mediated response in the host. They can develop through various mechanisms, including:

- retrovirus infection or other cause of cell transformation, which prompts production of a new protein.
- mutations that change protein structure. This occurs in major and minor histocompatibility antigens when chemical carcinogens induce tumors.
- exposure of normally unexposed antigenic determinants. For example, this occurs when a branch deleted from a complex glycolipid antigen reveals a new antigenic determinant.
- aberrant expression of fetal or differentiation antigens. For example, this occurs when ABO blood group antigens different from the host's ABO blood type appear on gastric carcinoma cells.

Types of tumor antigens. Tumor antigens can be divided into two types: tumor-specific and tumor-associated.

Tumor-specific antigens appear only on tumor cells and provide ideal targets for immunologic attack. Tumors induced by chemical carcinogens may express tumor-specific antigens.

Tumor-associated antigens (TAAs) appear on tumor cells and on some normal cells. Because TAAs differ from each other, they can be used to distinguish normal cells from tumor cells. These differences, revealed primarily by study of monoclonal antibodies, may include the amount of antigen expressed, its expression within a particular cell lineage, and differentiation markers.

Oncofetal antigens, the best understood TAAs, are expressed normally during fetal development. They're virtually absent in healthy adults, but appear in adults with certain tumors. For example, carcinoembryonic antigen (CEA), a glycoprotein normally found in the fetal gut, appears in colon cancer cells in adults. Shed from colon cancer cells and found in the serum, it helps in monitoring cancer patients' response to therapy. CEA, however, does not provide an effective cancer screening test, as originally thought, because it also appears in other tumors and lesions.

Continued on page 142

Tumor-related Immunologic Problems

Tumor growth—*continued*

Several other oncofetal antigens also have proved useful for monitoring tumors. Alpha-fetoprotein, normally secreted by fetal liver and yolk sac cells, appears in the serum of patients with hepatomas and germ cell tumors of the testis.

Differentiation and lineage-specific antigens, normally present on an adult's cells, may be aberrantly expressed on some tumor cells. For example, a T-cell antigen is commonly expressed on malignant B cells in chronic lymphocytic leukemia, and a red blood cell antigen appears on stomach cancer cells. These inappropriately expressed antigens help to identify tumor cells. Researchers have identified many other TAAs, but their function remains unknown. Tumor-associated molecules (TAMs) also appear on malignant cells; however, these molecules do not generate an immune response.

How the immune system responds to tumors
In the theory of *immunosurveillance,* the immune system surveys the body, recognizing and eventually destroying any immunogenic tumor cells that arise. Accordingly, a failure in immune function results in a malignancy. To lend credence to this theory, some researchers point to the high incidence of tumor growth in immunosuppressed patients. However, these patients don't experience an increase in all tumors, just lymphoreticular ones. As a result, researchers are modifying their views on immunosurveillance. They now think that antigen-specific responses probably play a part in preventing some tumors, especially those caused by oncogenic DNA and RNA viruses. Such effector populations as natural killer (NK) cells may also act in rejecting newly transformed cells.

In addition, immunosurveillance is probably not the only type of host surveillance that limits tumor development. Other local and systemic mechanisms maintain cells within tissues, sustain relationships between tissues during growth and development, and control repair and rejuvenation after injury.

Immune mechanisms and tumor cells
Every component of the immune system possesses the potential to eradicate tumor cells. These components include T cells, B cells, NK cells, and macrophages.

T cells. These cells play the most important role in controlling antigenic tumor cell growth. Two classes of T cells act on tumor cells: class I-restricted cells, which destroy tumor cells directly, and class II-restricted cells, which secrete lymphokines to activate other cells.

Because most tumor cells express class I but not class II antigens, the T-helper cells can't recognize these tumor cells. Instead, T-helper cells depend on such antigen-presenting cells as macrophages to present tumor antigens for activation. Once activated, T-helper cells secrete such lymphokines as interleukin-2 (IL-2), which in turn activate T-cytotoxic cells, macrophages, NK cells, and B cells. T-helper cells can produce other lymphokines, such as lymphotoxin or tumor necrosis factor, which may kill tumor cells directly. T-cytotoxic cells kill tumor cells by disrupting their membrane and

Tumor-related Immunologic Problems

nucleus. However, T-cytotoxic cells typically depend on T-helper responses to provide necessary helper factors to activate T-cytotoxic cell proliferation.

B cells. B cells, which contribute to antibody responses, appear in the serum when tumors are experimentally transplanted. What's more, spontaneous tumors may also elicit antibody responses to tumor-associated antigens. However, the importance of antibodies in controlling tumor growth isn't clear. For instance, a retrovirus can induce an antibody response that prevents development of tumors caused by that virus. But the antibody response does little to combat tumors that already exist. An effective response against a primary tumor requires an accompanying contribution by T cells. Nonetheless, antibodies that act weakly against the primary tumor may bind to circulating tumor cells and thwart metastasis.

Antibodies can destroy tumor cells in two ways. Complement-fixing antibodies bind to the tumor cell membrane, activate complement, and kill the cell. In antibody-dependent cell-mediated cytotoxicity, antibodies—usually IgG—form an intercellular bridge between the target cell and effector cells (macrophages, granulocytes, or killer cells).

NK cells. NK cells represent the first line of defense against the growth of tumor cells at both primary and metastatic sites. They also serve as effector cells that can be recruited by T cells to help supplement specific antitumor responses.

Just how NK cells recognize and destroy tumor cells isn't clear, but release of cytotoxic factor seems to occur and recognition doesn't seem to require binding to an antigen-specific receptor. Lymphokines—IL-2 and interferon—augment NK activity.

Additional cytotoxic effector cells include lymphokine-activated killer (LAK) cells, induced by high doses of IL-2. These differ from NK cells and attack a broader spectrum of tumor cells.

Macrophages. Macrophages act as antigen-presenting cells and as effector cells mediating tumor lysis. Macrophages become cytolytic to tumor cells through the action of macrophage-activating factor, a lymphokine secreted by T cells after antigen-specific stimulation. Precisely how activated macrophages recognize and attack tumors isn't fully understood.

Macrophages appear to be an important element in the antitumor effects of T-helper and T-cytotoxic cells. For instance, T-helper cells, which can't directly recognize most tumor cells, depend on activated effector cells like macrophages. T-cytotoxic cells, which do attack tumors directly, benefit from activated macrophages that supplement lysis. Macrophages may also eliminate potential variants in the tumor mass that no longer express antigenic determinants recognizable to T cells. (See *Steps in the immune response to tumor cells, page 144.)*

Although the immune system does respond to certain developing and established tumors, it doesn't respond to all tumors.

Continued on page 145

Tumor-related Immunologic Problems

Steps in the immune response to tumor cells

Step 1

Macrophages act as effector cells, engulfing tumor cells.

Macrophages also secrete alpha-interferon and interleukin-1 (IL-1). IL-1 activates T cells.

Step 2

T cells proliferate and produce gamma-interferon and interleukin-2 (IL-2).

Step 3

IL-2 promotes T-cell proliferation and growth and activates antigen-specific killer T cells.

Step 4

Gamma-interferon augments cell lysis by macrophages. Alpha-interferon augments natural killer (NK) cell activity.

Step 5

Lymphokine-activated killer (LAK) cells attack tumor cells and produce lymphotoxins that cause tumor cell lysis.

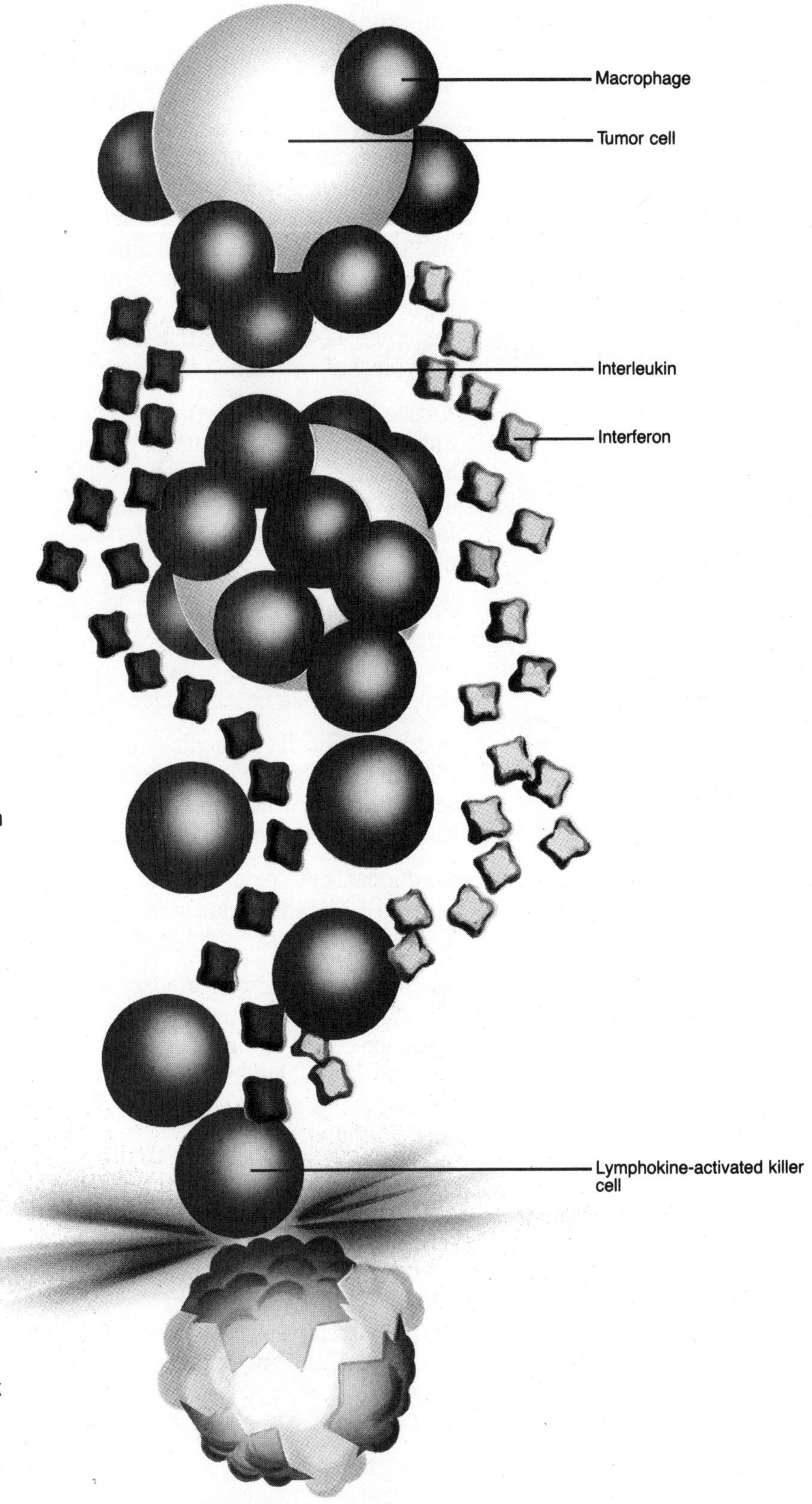

Tumor-related Immunologic Problems

Tumor growth—*continued*

How tumors escape the immune system

Besides the generalized immunodepression found in many cancer patients, various mechanisms allow tumor cells to circumvent or suppress a potentially threatening immune response. Immunologic escape occurs when the balance between factors favoring tumor growth and factors favoring tumor destruction tilts in favor of tumor growth. The following factors may contribute to immunologic escape:

Tumor kinetics. In early tumor development, when the number of tumor cells is small, the amount of antigen may not be sufficient to stimulate the immune system. This leads to tolerance. Subsequently, once tumor cells multiply sufficiently to trigger an immune response, their numbers may be too large to overcome.

Antigen modulation. In the presence of antibodies, some antigens are shed from the cell surface and redistributed within the cell membrane. This removal of target antigens recognizable to the immune system may allow the tumor to escape by making it less sensitive to the antibodies' cytotoxic effects.

Antigen masking. Tumors may escape from effector cells because such antigen-masking molecules as sialomucin bind to the tumor cell surface and mask the tumor antigens, preventing adhesion of attacking lymphocytes. Antigen masking can be reversed by therapy aimed at degrading antigen-masking molecules.

Antigen shedding. Circulating soluble tumor antigens may compromise cell-mediated immunity by saturating antigen-binding sites. A similar paralysis of the local effector response can be produced by antigen-antibody (immune) complexes.

Tolerance. The normal immune response to tumor antigens may be inhibited.

Lymphocyte trapping. Tumor-specific lymphocytes may be trapped in lymph nodes draining the tumor. In these nodes, local lymphocytes may become tolerant of the tumor antigen, while lymphocytes at distant sites remain unaffected and react normally to antigens.

Genetic factors. Patients with certain major histocompatibility complex (MHC) haplotypes may fail to induce an effector T-cell response to a tumor, probably because of the MHC's inability to form a suitable associated complex with the foreign antigen. In fact, some tumors express no Class I antigens at all.

Blocking factors. Once shed, tumor cell antigens may form complexes with the host's specific antibodies. These complexes could block host T lymphocytes in two ways:
- by binding directly to T-cytotoxic cells, preventing them from engaging tumor cells
- by binding to T-helper cells, preventing them from recognizing the tumor and assisting T-cytotoxic cells.

Also, if antibodies induced by the shed antigens aren't effective, they could bind antigens on tumor cells and prevent T-helper cells

Continued on page 146

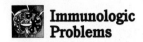

Tumor-related Immunologic Problems

Tumor growth—*continued*

and T-cytotoxic cells from engaging the tumor. Even if antibodies have the potential to kill the tumor, shed antigens may bind to the antitumor antibodies before they reach their target, rendering the antibodies ineffective.

Tumor products. Nonantigen tumor products may interfere with the immune response. Prostaglandins, for example, negatively affect NK-cell and K-cell function. Other humoral factors impair the inflammatory response, chemotaxis, and the complement cascade. They also promote formation of a blood supply within solid tumors.

Growth factors. Interleukins are essential to amplifying T-cell responses. Reduced macrophage production of interleukin-1 (IL-1), diminished cooperation between T-cell subsets, or limited availability of IL-2 could limit overall response to a tumor.

The fact that many tumors escape doesn't necessarily invalidate the theory of immunosurveillance. If immunosurveillance exists, it probably depends on a balance between mechanisms that reduce tumor viability, immune escape, and immunodepression.

Tumor immunodiagnosis

Tumor immunodiagnosis refers to the use of tumor antigens, along with the products of the immune system's response to tumors, to help diagnose tumors and monitor response to therapy. These techniques developed from such scientific advances as recombinant DNA technology and hybridoma technology (monoclonal antibodies).

Tumor markers

Tumor cells express cell-surface, cytoplasmic, and secreted products that differ from those produced by normal cells. These products function as tumor markers—biological indicators that help detect the presence of a tumor. Most tumor markers are actually normal products found in abnormal concentrations or products that are normally present during development but not during adult life.

Following tumor ablation, serum levels of these markers decline. Increasing serum levels may provide an early indication of disease recurrence or the patient's failure to respond to therapy. Tumor markers also help determine prognosis. (See *Applications of tumor markers.*)

Tumor markers can be divided into two categories: tumor-derived and tumor-associated. *Tumor-derived* markers are produced by tumor cells and include:

- Hormones—antidiuretic hormone, calcitonin, catecholamines and metabolites, human chorionic gonadotropin, insulin-like growth factors, parathyroid hormone
- Oncofetal antigens—alpha-fetoprotein, carcinoembryonic antigen
- Isoenzymes—lactic dehydrogenase-1, neuron-specific enolase, prostatic acid phosphatase, regan alkaline phosphatase
- Oncogenes and related products—H-ras, N-myc, src

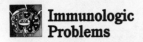

Tumor-related Immunologic Problems

• Tissue-specific proteins—alpha-lactalbumin, $beta_2$-microglobulin, immunoglobulins, prostate-specific antigen, tumor-associated antigen
• Mucins and other glycoproteins—CA-15-3, CA-19-9, CA-125
• Other tumor-derived markers—glycolipids, polyamines, sialic acid.

Tumor-associated markers are produced by normal tissue in response to a tumor. Because these substances are indicators of immune activation, they may respond to a tumor or a nontumorigenic stimulus, and therefore do not specifically indicate cancer. But when used with tumor-derived markers, tumor-associated markers provide additional information for determining or confirming the progress of certain cancers, thereby aiding in therapeutic management. They include:
• acute phase proteins
• ferritin
• immune complexes
• isoenzymes.

Tumor-associated markers under investigation include:
• IL-2 receptors
• tumor necrosis factor or cachectin
• neopterin.
(For information on tumor markers and the cancers they help detect, see *Tumor markers and their associated cancers* below.)

Continued on page 148

Applications of tumor markers

Two new tumor markers may detect cancer of any type or clinical stage.

The first is an antibody tumor marker, which has been approved by the Food and Drug Administration. The second tumor marker, still investigational, uses nuclear magnetic resonance (NMR) spectroscopy to examine plasma lipids.

Anti-malignin antibody test
A valuable diagnostic tool for patients with cancer symptoms, this test measures the amount of anti-malignin antibody. This antibody increases threefold to tenfold in a patient with any type of cancer. The test produces few false-positive findings and doesn't depend on the type or stage of cancer.

NMR spectroscopy
This procedure analyzes spectral patterns of plasma lipids and can detect a characteristic abnormality in certain lipoproteins of cancer patients. By alerting doctors to the possibility of cancer somewhere in the patient's body, the test may help pinpoint a specific cancer months or years before symptoms appear. What's more, it may help monitor the effectiveness of cancer treatments.

Tumor markers and their associated cancers

Marker	Associated cancers
COMMON TUMOR MARKERS	
Alpha-fetoprotein	Liver, testis
CA-125	Ovary
Calcitonin	Medullary cancer of thyroid
Carcinoembryonic antigen	Colon, lung, breast
Human chorionic gonadotropin	Trophoblastic tumors, germ cell tumors of testis
Immunoglobulins	Multiple myeloma
Prostatic acid phosphatase	Prostate
INVESTIGATIONAL TUMOR MARKERS	
CA-15-3	Breast
CA-19-9	Pancreas, colon
Creatine kinase BB isoenzyme	Lung, breast, prostate
Lactate dehydrogenase-1	Testis
Neuron-specific enolase	Small-cell carcinoma of the lung, neuroblastoma
Prostate-specific antigen	Prostate
Tumor-associated antigen	Uterine, cervix

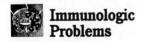

Tumor-related Immunologic Problems

Tumor immunotherapy

Cancer therapies exploit the differences between normal cells and tumor cells. These therapies take a number of approaches: anatomic (surgery and radiation therapy), metabolic (chemotherapy), cell cycle kinetics (radiation therapy and chemotherapy), and antigenic (immune responses). (See *Types of tumor immunotherapy*.) Therapies that use immunologic or biological agents are collectively termed *biological response modifiers* (BRMs).

BRMs alter the relationship between tumor and host by modifying the host's biological response to tumor cells. BRMs are classified into three categories:

- immunomodulation, where the agents restore, augment, or modulate the host's immune system
- direct activity, where agents have direct antitumor effects
- other biological effects, where agents interfere with a tumor cell's ability to metastasize or survive, or affect cell transformation. (See *How BRMs act against tumors*.)

The way BRMs work is not fully understood. Some agents possess more than one antitumor mechanism. Although BRMs work mainly through the immune system, they do achieve some effects through other systems as well. Important BRMs include interferon, IL-2, and monoclonal antibodies.

Interferon

Interferon refers to a variety of natural and recombinant lymphokines that work by active immune mechanisms. (See *Sources of interferon*, page 150, and *Producing interferon*, page 151.) Interferon performs three major functions:

Viral inhibition. Interferon inhibits DNA replication in a virus that has invaded a cell. At the same time, interferon protects the infected cell from invasion by other viruses.

Immunomodulation. Interferon interacts with T cells to stimulate the creation of cellular products that signal monocytes, NK cells, and other T cells to recognize and destroy tumor cells.

Antiproliferative or antitumor effects. Just how interferon achieves these effects isn't clear. It may attack the tumor directly, augment or induce immune recognition of the tumor, or induce membrane antigens on tumor cells, thereby allowing subsequent immune recognition.

The three major classes of interferon are: alpha-interferon (derived from leukocytes), beta-interferon (derived from fibroblasts), and gamma-interferon (derived from lymphocytes). Recombinant alpha-interferon has been approved by the Food and Drug Administration (FDA) for use in hairy-cell leukemia. Besides hairy-cell leukemia, tumors that respond to alpha-interferon therapy include chronic myelogenous leukemia, non-Hodgkin's lymphoma, cutaneous T-cell lymphoma, Kaposi's sarcoma, renal cell carcinoma, and mycosis fungoides. Researchers are also exploring the use of alpha-interferon therapy combined with other lymphokines or with conventional therapy (such as chemotherapy). Alpha-interferon's antiviral effects

Tumor-related Immunologic Problems

How BRMs act against tumors

Biological response modifiers (BRMs) include several types of agents that can be used in immunotherapy.

Immunomodulatory agents include:
- alpha-, beta-, and gamma-interferons
- interferon inducers, such as *Sendai* virus
- lymphokines, such as interleukin-2 and gamma-interferon
- nonspecific immunomodulatory agents, such as bacille Calmette-Guérin and *Corynebacterium parvum*
- tumor cells used in active, specific immunizations.

Directly cytotoxic or cytostatic agents include:
- adoptive immunotherapeutic agents, such as lymphokine-activated killer cells
- interferon and interferon inducers
- tumor necrosis factor.

Other agents include:
- colony stimulating factor
- differentiating agents, such as growth factors and retinoids
- metastasis preventors, such as laminin and anticoagulants.

Types of tumor immunotherapy

Immunotherapy can be divided into two types, active and passive. *Active* immunotherapy induces an immune response to a tumor, whereas *passive* or *adoptive* immunotherapy transfers to the host immunologically active reagents that mediate a response.

Active	Passive
Active immunotherapies may be specific or nonspecific. Specific therapies include: • autologous and allogeneic inactivated tumor vaccines • human tumor hybrids (with xenogeneic antigen-bearing fusion partners) • monoclonal tumor anti-idiotypic antibodies. Nonspecific therapies include: • biological immunostimulants, such as bacille Calmette-Guérin (BCG), methanol-extracted BCG residue, cyclophosphamide, *Corynebacterium parvum,* and OK-432 • chemical immunostimulants, such as levamisole, picabanyl, cimetidine, and lysosomes containing macrophage-activating substances • chemotherapeutic drugs, such as cyclophosphamide, melphalan, cisplatin, doxorubicin, and vinca alkaloids • cytokines, such as interferon, interleukin-2, and tumor necrosis factor.	Passive immunotherapies also may be specific or nonspecific. Specific therapies include: • allogeneic bone marrow transplants accompanied by chemotherapy or radiation therapy • autologous, allogeneic, or xenographic T cells • heterologous antiserum from immunized human donors • monoclonal antibodies, including murine, human, and chimeric • monoclonal lymphocytes from T cells. Nonspecific therapies include: • activated macrophages, such as interferon and phorbol esters • cytostatic or cytotoxic cytokines, such as interferon and tumor necrosis factor • lymphocyte-activated killer cells generated by interleukin.

are being used against the papovavirus that causes genital and laryngeal warts. (See *Alpha-interferon and multiple sclerosis*, page 151.)

Tumors most responsive to beta- and gamma-interferons include melanoma, sarcoma, breast cancer, renal cancer, and lymphoid malignancies. Gamma-interferon alters lipid metabolism and activates monocytes, thereby reducing tumor growth. It exerts a synergistic effect with tumor necrosis factor (cachectin), another recombinant lymphokine, in stimulating regulatory molecules.

Nursing considerations. When administering interferon, keep in mind that the drug is manufactured by recombinant-DNA technology and differs in stability among subtypes, dilutions, diluents, and batches. Its effects differ depending on whether it is human interferon, which includes several subtypes, or cloned interferon, which consists of only one purified protein.

Always check the manufacturer's instructions to verify correct dosage, concentration, recommended route of administration, reconstitution, and stability of each brand of interferon. Usually, you'll give interferon S.C. or I.V., but remember that the administration route affects serum levels and therefore influences therapeutic and adverse effects. Interferon is measured in units of antiviral activity (its ability to inhibit viral replication in tissue culture); typical measurement is by the megaunit, which equals one million units.

Continued on page 150

Tumor-related Immunologic Problems

Sources of interferon

Type	Subtype	Source
Alpha	Leukocyte (IFN alpha [Le])	Leukocytes from normal blood
	Lymphoblastoid (IFN alfa-N1)	Lymphoblastoid (Namalva) cells in culture
	Recombinant alpha-2 (interferon alfa-2b)	Transformed *Escherichia coli*
	Recombinant alpha-A (interferon alfa-2a)	Transformed *E. coli*
	Recombinant alpha-D (interferon alfa-D)	Transformed *E. coli*
Beta	Fibroblast (interferon beta)	Fetal foreskin fibroblasts in culture
	Recombinant beta-cys	Transformed *E. coli*
	Recombinant beta-ser	Transformed *E. coli*
Gamma	Immune	T cells from normal blood
	Recombinant gamma	Transformed *E. coli*

Tumor immunotherapy—*continued*

Watch for these adverse reactions to interferon:

• *Flulike syndrome.* Chills, fever, malaise, and myalgias lasting 5 to 9 days occur in 90% of patients receiving a first dose greater than 1 megaunit/m². Chills usually begin 3 to 6 hours after administration and include shivering, teeth-chattering rigors, and pallor induced by vasoconstriction. If the patient received high doses of interferon, he may require morphine to thwart severe muscle contractions if rigors last more than 10 minutes. Fever usually peaks at 102° to 104° F. (39° to 40° C.) about an hour after onset of chills.

Typically, you can control fever by giving acetaminophen before interferon administration and every 3 to 4 hours afterward. Don't give aspirin, nonsteroidal anti-inflammatory drugs, or corticosteroids because they may block enzyme production, hindering interferon's effectiveness. Try to administer interferon in the late afternoon or evening so that the fever occurs before bedtime. Many patients will sleep through the discomfort, although they may awaken tired and sore.

Although the patient's flulike signs and symptoms may suggest infection, you'll be able to identify them as drug effects because the pattern is predictable: symptoms occur within a specified time, last for a limited period, and respond to acetaminophen.

The patient may also experience muscle aches, headache, fatigue, generalized malaise, and a low-grade fever for up to 20 hours after the first dose.

• *Chronic fatigue.* This symptom usually worsens during the course of therapy, especially if the patient receives high doses of interferon. Prepare the patient for this so he doesn't assume that his disease has worsened. Also, help him to plan rest periods.

Continued on page 152

Tumor-related Immunologic Problems

Alpha-interferon and multiple sclerosis

A recent study indicates that natural alpha-interferon therapy may have long-term benefits for patients with early and mild relapsing multiple sclerosis (MS). According to the study, alpha-interferon enabled MS patients to perform normal daily activities. Overall neurologic function, however, didn't change significantly. Researchers do not know the precise mechanism of this beneficial effect but believe it involves immunoregulatory functions.

Producing interferon

Steps in the production of interferon by recombinant-DNA technology include:

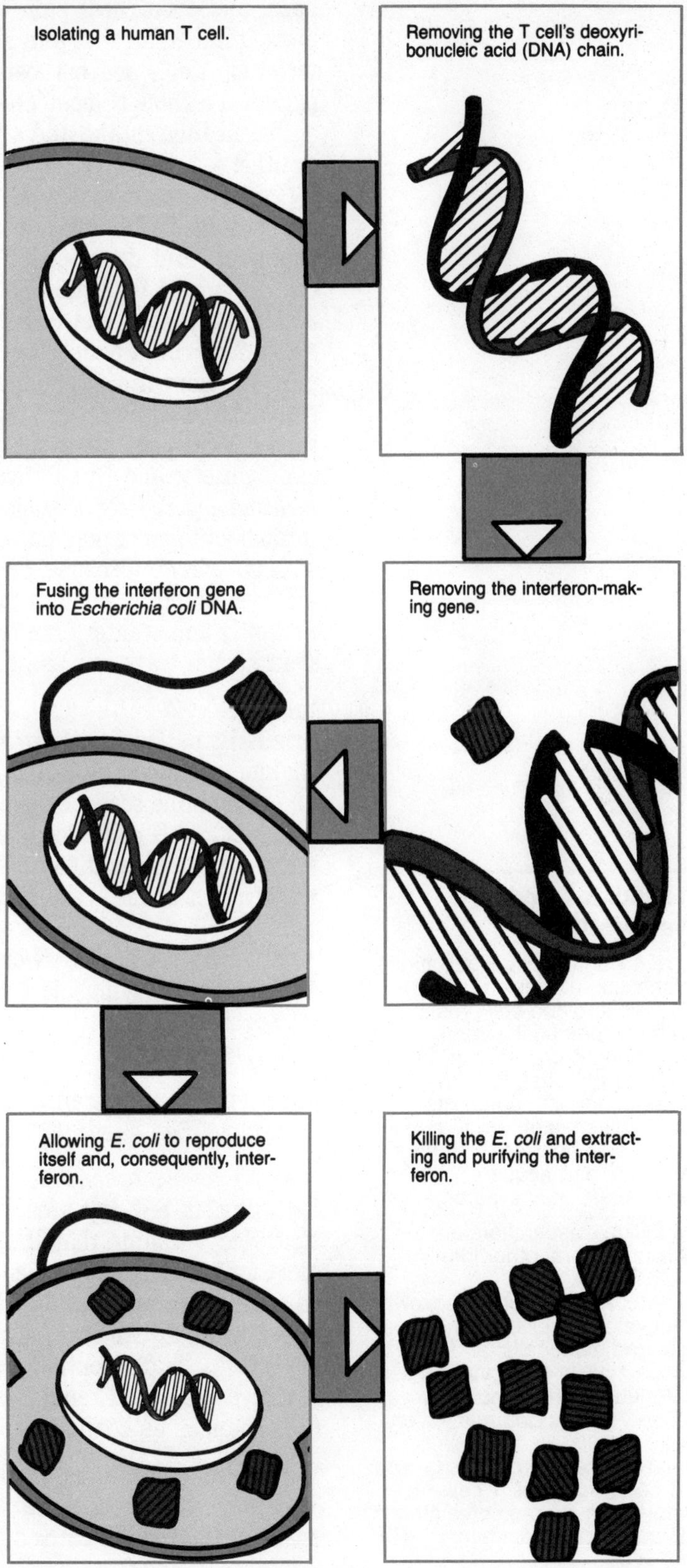
Isolating a human T cell.
Removing the T cell's deoxyribonucleic acid (DNA) chain.
Removing the interferon-making gene.
Fusing the interferon gene into *Escherichia coli* DNA.
Allowing *E. coli* to reproduce itself and, consequently, interferon.
Killing the *E. coli* and extracting and purifying the interferon.

Tumor-related Immunologic Problems

Tumor immunotherapy—*continued*

• *Cardiovascular effects.* Symptoms may appear during acute flulike episodes. Assess patients for pallor, tachycardia, cyanosis, tachypnea, and even chest pain with nonspecific EKG changes. Rarely, myocardial infarction and sudden death occur after receiving interferon. You'll see orthostatic hypotension in two out of three patients, although most don't notice it. Manage this by ensuring sufficient fluid intake and avoiding sudden changes in the patient's position.
• *Central nervous system (CNS) effects.* CNS toxicity can occur at any dosage. With low doses, you may find the patient irritable, impatient, and depressed. With moderate doses, you may detect confusion and forgetfulness. With high doses, you may find the patient paranoiac and fearful of impending doom.
• *GI effects.* Mild nausea occurs during the first week of treatment in about one third of patients receiving moderate doses; it usually responds to antiemetics. Diarrhea occasionally occurs; vomiting, rarely. More commonly, the patient will complain of altered taste, early satiety, and cumulative anorexia.
• *Hematologic effects.* Transient, mild granulocytopenia; anemia; and thrombocytopenia may occur.
• *Renal effects.* Because interferon is excreted primarily by the kidneys, carefully monitor patients with preexisting renal disease. Promptly adjust interferon dosage, if needed. Proteinuria and transient serum transaminase elevations may occur.

Interleukin-2
Originally called T-cell growth factor, interleukin-2 (IL-2) is a lymphokine produced by stimulated T cells. IL-2 plays an important role in immune response because it stimulates T cells, B cells, NK cells, and LAK cells. Its effects include:
• lymphoid proliferation and reversal of immune deficiency
• activation of the lytic mechanisms of LAK cells and T-cytolytic cells
• enhanced effect of LAK or specific antitumor T cells
• emigration of lymphoid cells from peripheral blood into tissues
• release of various other lymphokines, including gamma-interferon, and other hormones, including growth hormone.

Patients with renal cell carcinoma and melanoma benefit from IL-2 therapy. (See *Interleukins under investigation*.)

Nursing considerations. Administer IL-2 by I.V. bolus, continuous I.V. infusion, S.C. injection, or intrahepatic or intraperitoneal infusion. Keep in mind that IL-2 affects every major body system. Be alert for common adverse effects: a flulike syndrome that includes nausea, vomiting, and diarrhea (treated with acetaminophen, indomethacin, antiemetics, and antidiarrheals); a marked cutaneous erythema; fluid retention; eosinophilia; anemia; and moderate to severe hepatic and renal dysfunction. You may also observe such CNS changes as confusion, disorientation, psychosis, and anxiety.

You may also encounter capillary-leak syndrome with IL-2 therapy. This may occur from extravasation of fluids into the extravascular space or fluid shifts caused by eosinophilia. When IL-2 is stopped,

Interleukins under investigation

Currently under investigation, the lymphokine interleukin-3 (IL-3) spurs white blood cell production and holds potential as an infection-fighting drug. Scientists hope to use IL-3 to ease the adverse effects on the immune system caused by chemotherapy, radiation therapy, bone marrow transplantation, and acquired immunodeficiency syndrome.

In addition, researchers are studying several other interleukins:
• Interleukin-4—promotes growth of activated B cells, resting T cells, and mast cells; and enhances activity of T-cytolytic cells
• Interleukin-5—promotes growth of T and B cells and maturation of eosinophils
• Interleukin-6—promotes growth of B cells, activates T cells
• Interleukin-7—promotes growth of B and T cell progenitors.

Tumor-related Immunologic Problems

Lymphokine-activated killer cells

Interleukin-2 (IL-2) can turn peripheral lymphocytes into lymphokine-activated killer (LAK) cells that attack cancer cells but leave normal cells unharmed. Adoptive immunotherapy that combines infusions of LAK cells with IL-2 may help patients with melanoma, non-Hodgkin's lymphoma, and colorectal cancer. It can, however, cause minor adverse effects, such as headache, fever, chills, and nausea.

Apparently, LAK-cell precursor lymphocytes are null cells, which require IL-2 activation before they can generate LAK cells. Before therapy begins, LAK cell precursors are collected from the patient by leukapheresis, separated out, and incubated with IL-2 to intensify LAK production. Then the new LAK cells are washed and resuspended in a normal saline and 5% serum albumin solution for reinfusion.

To maintain LAK cell activity, first infuse both IL-2 and the LAK cells as ordered. Then stop the LAK-cell infusion and continue to infuse IL-2 for several more days to prompt continued LAK production. When the IL-2 infusion stops, LAK production also stops.

This therapy has various benefits:
- IL-2 appears more effective when given with LAK cells.
- Using IL-2 to provoke the body to create LAK cells is more effective than just infusing LAK cells.
- LAK cells are easily generated and apparently tumor-specific. They also exhibit broad, cell-killing activity.
- The therapy doesn't depend on immunocompetence and may supplement immunosuppressive therapies. It's also effective in many types of cancer.

Another form of therapy currently under investigation combines IL-2 with tumor-infiltrating lymphocytes (TILs). TILs are killer T cells. Like LAK cells, they attack cancer cells; however, they appear to be much more potent.

this third-space shift reverses quickly, and you may observe vasodilation and hypotension. (See *Adverse effects of interleukin-2 therapy,* page 154.)

When given with LAK cells, IL-2 may cause marked hypotension, reflecting a reduction in systemic vascular resistance. The patient may require vasopressors. (See *Lymphokine-activated killer cells.*)

Most toxicities relate directly to dosage and symptoms usually resolve within 96 hours after stopping IL-2. However, some patients report malaise, flulike symptoms, skin desquamation, anorexia, taste changes, and peripheral edema for 2 to 3 weeks following therapy.

Monoclonal antibodies

Technological developments now allow reproduction of monoclonal antibodies (also called MoAbs) in almost unlimited quantities. Almost all of these are murine antibodies against human antigens, produced by mouse B-cell hybridomas. (See *Creation of monoclonal antibodies,* page 155.)

In cancer therapies, cytotoxic monoclonal antibodies have been used. Other monoclonal antibodies that have been used in cancer therapies can:
- join with a drug or other agent to deliver a cytotoxic agent to tumors
- render a tumor unable to divide or survive
- mirror tumor-cell antigens and stimulate antitumor activity.

Monoclonal antibodies have been used in clinical trials for treatment of acute T-cell leukemia, B-cell lymphoma, melanoma, and colon carcinoma. (See *Monoclonal antibodies and their antitumor effects,* page 155.) Monoclonal antibodies can also be used for:
- blood typing
- differentiating subpopulations of B cells and T cells
- monitoring organ graft rejection
- detecting pregnancy as early as nine days after conception
- detecting pathogens earlier than previously possible
- diagnosing diseases that are difficult to identify.

Monoclonal antibodies are also being tested for use in:
- preventing graft-versus-host disease
- purging leukemic cells from bone marrow in autologous transplants
- treating acute renal transplant rejection
- developing new drug assays
- treating drug toxicity.

Nursing considerations. You'll usually administer monoclonal antibodies by slow I.V. infusion over 1 or 2 hours. The length of the infusion time varies depending on the dose and whether the purpose is diagnostic or therapeutic. You also may give them by hepatic intraarterial infusion when treating liver metastases.

Monoclonal antibodies cause relatively few adverse effects. Those that do occur often stem from allergic reaction to the mouse protein from which monoclonal antibodies are refined. This reaction includes fever, chills, headache, flushing, urticaria, rash, dyspnea, hypoten-

Continued on page 154

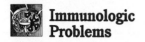

Tumor-related Immunologic Problems

Tumor immunotherapy—*continued*

sion, tachycardia, and anaphylactic or anaphylactoid reactions. Watch patients who receive multiple infusions. Their risk of experiencing an allergic reaction rises with each infusion.

Other biological response modifiers
Other BRMs under investigation for tumor immunotherapy include immunomodulating agents (immunopotentiation agents), hematologic growth factors, and other lymphokines (cytokines).

Adverse effects of interleukin-2 therapy

Patients undergoing interleukin-2 (IL-2) therapy may develop a variety of adverse effects. Watch patients for the following signs and symptoms:

Dermatologic effects

The patient may experience erythematous rash, pruritus, and skin desquamation. The cause is unknown. Interventions may include:
- administering prophylactic diphenhydramine (Benadryl)
- assessing skin daily
- applying water-based lotion or cream to skin twice daily
- instructing the patient to avoid scrubbing and to pat skin dry after bathing.

Gastrointestinal effects

The patient may suffer from nausea, vomiting, diarrhea, mucositis, or loss of appetite. The cause is unknown. Interventions may include:
- monitoring intake and output during infusion and the following day
- administering prophylactic antiemetics and antidiarrheal agents, as ordered
- assessing oral mucosa daily
- advising the patient to eat more frequent, smaller meals each day.

Hematologic effects

Hematologic effects, such as anemia and thrombocytopenia, are related to cumulative IL-2 levels. Interventions may include:
- monitoring complete blood count daily. If platelet count falls under 65,000/mm^3, avoid rectal suppositories, rectal thermometers, and I.M. injections.
- assessing for petechiae, bruising, or bleeding gums
- testing stool, urine, and emesis for blood.

Neurologic effects

Neurologic effects may include confusion, disorientation, combativeness, psychosis, and anxiety. Scientists have not established the cause of these effects; they may result from sleep deprivation or the stress of intensive care. Interventions may include:
- assessing the patient's neurologic status before therapy
- observing for central nervous system metastases
- observing for personality changes
- educating the patient and his family. Explain that symptoms may be dose-related and that you may have to interrupt or stop IL-2 treatments. Explain also that adverse effects are reversible.
- taking steps to assure patient safety.

Pulmonary and cardiovascular effects

Reduced systemic vascular resistance may lead to hypotension. Possible interventions include:
- monitoring vital signs
- administering 5% albumin, dopamine, or phenylephrine to maintain systolic blood pressure above 100 mm Hg.

Patients may also experience weight gain, peripheral or pulmonary edema, ascites, dysrhythmias, or dyspnea. These symptoms are caused by increased capillary permeability and extravasation of fluid into extravascular space or fluid shifts due to eosinophilia. Possible interventions include:
- monitoring fluid intake and output
- weighing patient daily
- measuring abdominal girth in patients with ascites
- elevating extremities in patients with peripheral edema
- observing for shortness of breath or altered breathing.

Renal effects

The patient may experience oliguria, proteinuria, and elevated creatinine or blood urea nitrogen (BUN) levels. IL-2 acts directly on kidneys, with the effect related to cumulative levels. Interventions may include:
- monitoring the patient's intake and output during infusion and the following day
- monitoring BUN, creatinine, and urine protein levels.

Other adverse effects

Fever following administration of IL-2 may be the result of direct action on the hypothalamic centers. Alternatively, IL-2 may stimulate other lymphokines that act on the hypothalamus. Possible interventions include:
- administering acetaminophen prophylactically
- monitoring temperature, both during infusion and the following day
- providing the patient with a cooling mattress.

Patients may experience chills or rigors. Administer meperidine, as ordered.

Patients may also experience headache, malaise, flulike syndrome, nasal congestion, glossitis, or xerostomia. The cause of these adverse effects remains unknown. If symptoms persist after the patient leaves the hospital, advise him to rest and continue taking acetaminophen.

Tumor-related Immunologic Problems

Monoclonal antibodies and their antitumor effects

Antibody	Tumor
Leu1 (Anti-CD5)	T-cell lymphoma
Anti-idiotype	B-cell lymphoma
17-1A	Gastrointestinal carcinoma
R24 (Anti-GD3 Ganglioside)	Melanoma
L72 (Anti-GD2 Ganglioside; Human IgM)	Melanoma
XMMME (001) Ricin-A-conjugate	Melanoma
3 F8 (Anti-GD2 Ganglioside)	Melanoma, neuroblastoma

Creation of monoclonal antibodies

Creation of monoclonal antibodies starts with injection of a desired antigen into a mouse. After injection, the mouse begins producing antibody-secreting B cells in response to the antigen. Next, B cells are removed from the mouse's spleen and combined with myeloma (or other) cells from a second mouse. Then a fusion agent, such as polyethylene glycol, is added to the cells.

Some B cells hybridize with some of the myeloma cells, resulting in antibody-secreting cells that are virtually immortal. Next, these antibody-secreting cells are then cloned in culture or in a third mouse. Purified monoclonal antibodies can then be gathered from the tissue culture's supernatant fluid or from the mouse's ascitic fluid.

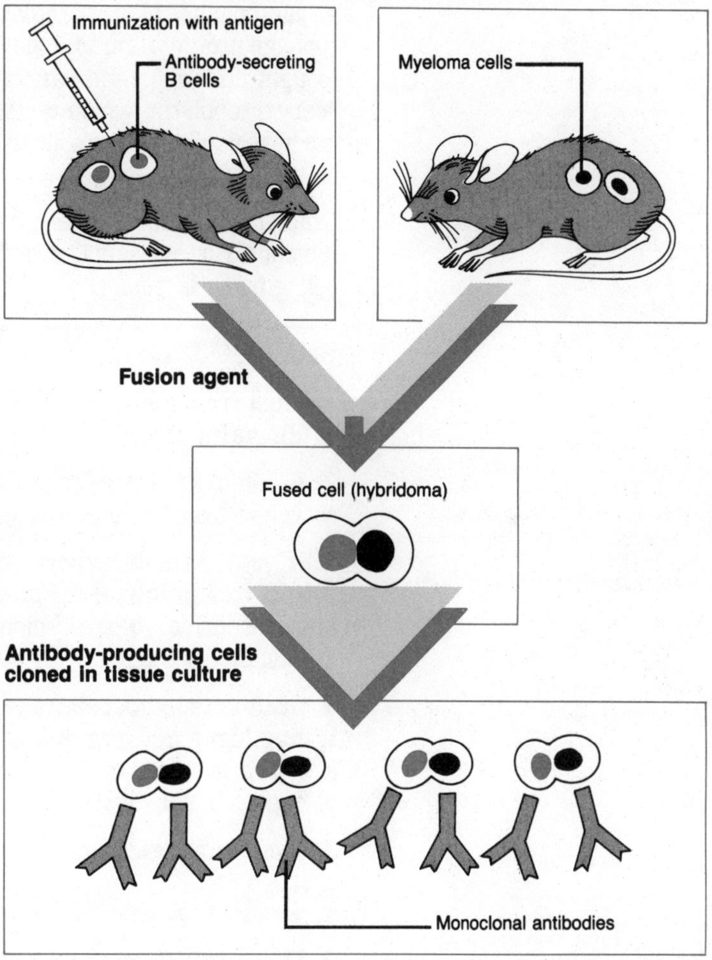

Immunomodulating agents. These agents modify the immune system or its components in an effort to control or destroy cancerous cells. They include adjuvants, which enhance the immune response when injected along with an antigen. Adjuvants increase the surface area of an antigen or prolong its retention in the body. Adjuvants may also expand T-cell and B-cell populations.

Nonspecific immunomodulating agents include bacille Calmette-Guérin (BCG), *Corynebacterium parvum*, polyinosinic-polycytidylic acid (poly I:C), polyadenylic-polyuridylic acid (poly A:U), levamisole, bestatin, lentinan, muramyldipeptide (MTP-PE), OK-432, and PSK. Specific immunomodulating agents include the immunogenic RNAs and transfer factor.

Continued on page 156

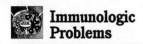

Tumor-related Immunologic Problems

Tumor immunotherapy—*continued*

Hematologic growth factors. These agents boost immune responses and stimulate the growth of red and white blood cells. These natural hormones include:

- granulocyte colony stimulating factor (G-CSF), which increases neutrophil activity. It may help treat infections and cancer and aid in bone marrow transplantation
- granulocyte-macrophage colony stimulating factor (GM-CSF), which enhances production of macrophages, neutrophils, eosinophils, and possibly red blood cells
- macrophage colony stimulating factor (M-CSF), which causes macrophage proliferation and may trigger GM-CSF production; it seems to fight infections and cancer
- erythropoietin, which is necessary for erythropoiesis. Researchers have used this hormone to treat anemia; it also helps to replenish blood during surgery.

Other lymphokines. These agents include tumor necrosis factor, lymphotoxin, epidermal growth factor, tumor growth factor, and B-cell growth factor.

Self-Test

1. Most transplanted grafts are:
a. allografts **b.** autografts **c.** syngrafts **d.** xenografts

2. A common sign of transplant rejection is:
a. weight loss **b.** hypertension **c.** low-grade fever **d.** anuria

3. If your patient experiences a transplant rejection, you can expect to administer all of the following except:
a. cyclosporine **b.** antilymphocyte globulin **c.** azathioprine **d.** immune globulin

4. Graft-versus-host disease may be staged using all of the following signs and symptoms except:
a. type and extent of skin rash **b.** amount of weight loss **c.** degree of hyperbilirubinemia **d.** amount of diarrhea

5. The carcinogens most likely to activate the immune system are:
a. chemical **b.** physical **c.** viral **d.** environmental

6. These cells play the most important role in controlling tumor cell growth:
a. T cells **b.** B cells **c.** NK cells **d.** macrophages

7. If a patient receiving interferon develops fever, expect to administer:
a. acetaminophen **b.** aspirin **c.** nonsteroidal anti-inflammatory drugs **d.** corticosteroids

8. Capillary-leak syndrome may occur with administration of:
a. alpha-interferon **b.** interleukin-2 **c.** monoclonal antibodies **d.** gamma-interferon

Answers (page number shows where answer appears in text)
1. **a** (page 122) 2. **c** (page 126) 3. **d** (page 131) 4. **b** (page 135) 5. **c** (page 140) 6. **a** (page 142) 7. **a** (page 150) 8. **b** (page 152)

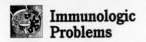

Selected References

Books

Bellanti, J. *Immunology III.* Philadelphia: W.B. Saunders Co., 1985.

Bobak, I., and Jensen, M. *Essentials of Maternity Nursing,* 2nd ed. St. Louis: C.V. Mosby Co., 1987.

Cerilli, G. *Organ Transplantation and Replacement.* Philadelphia: J.B. Lippincott Co., 1988.

Griffin, J. *Hematology and Immunology: Concepts for Nursing.* East Norwalk, Conn.: Appleton & Lange, 1986.

Groenwald, S. *Cancer Nursing: Principles and Practices.* Boston: Jones and Bartlett Pubs., Inc., 1987.

Guyton, A. *Textbook of Medical Physiology.* Philadelphia: W.B. Saunders Co., 1986.

Lahita, R., ed. *Systemic Lupus Erythematosus.* New York: John Wiley & Sons, 1987.

Lichtenstein, L., and Fauci, A., eds. *Current Therapy in Allergy, Immunology, and Rheumatology.* St. Louis: C.V. Mosby Co., 1985.

Porth, C. *Pathophysiology.* Philadelphia: J.B. Lippincott Co., 1986.

Roitt, I., et al. *Immunology.* St. Louis: C.V. Mosby Co., 1985.

Smolen, J., and Zielinski, C., eds. *Systemic Lupus Erythematosus: Clinical and Experimental Aspects.* New York: Springer-Verlag, 1987.

Stites, D., et al., eds. *Basic and Clinical Immunology.* East Norwalk, Conn.: Appleton & Lange, 1987.

Periodicals

Abernathy, E. "Biotherapy: An Introductory Overview," *Oncology Nursing Forum Supplement* 14(6):13-15, November/December 1987.

Abernathy, E. "Immunology: How the Immune System Works," and "Immunology: Biological Response Modifiers," *American Journal of Nursing* 87(4):456-59, April 1987.

American Cancer Society. "Immunology and Cancer," *Ca-A Cancer Journal for Clinicians* 38(2):66-128, March/April 1988.

Bach, F., and Sachs, D. "Transplant Immunology," *New England Journal of Medicine* 317(8):489-92, August 1987.

Barbour, S. "Acquired Immunodeficiency Syndrome of Childhood," *Pediatric Clinics of North America* 34(1):247-68, January/February 1987.

Buckley, R. "Immunodeficiency Diseases," *Journal of the American Medical Association* 258(20):2841-49, November 1987.

Centers for Disease Control. *Morbidity and Mortality Weekly Report* 36 (1S and 2S), August 1987.

Condemi, J. "The Autoimmune Diseases," *Journal of the American Medical Association* 258(20):2920-29, November 1987.

Creticos, P., and Phillips, N. "Immunotherapy with Allergens," *Journal of the American Medical Association* 258(20):2874-80, November 1987.

Dinarello, C., and Mier, J. "Current Concepts—Lymphokines," *New England Journal of Medicine* 317(15):940-45, October 1987.

Friedland, G., and Klein, R. "Transmission of the Human Immunodeficiency Virus," *New England Journal of Medicine* 317(18):1125-33, October 1987.

Gallucci, B. "The Immune System and Cancer," *Oncology Nursing Forum Supplement* 14(6):3-12, November/December 1987.

Ho, D., et al. "Pathogenesis of Infection with Human Immunodeficiency Virus," *New England Journal of Medicine* 317(5):278-83, July 1987.

Hood, L. "Biological Response Modifiers: Interferon," *American Journal of Nursing* 87(4):459-64, April 1987.

Jassak, P., and Spiewak, P. "Immunology: Interleukin-2," *American Journal of Nursing* 87(4):464-67, April 1987.

Kirpatrick, C. "Transplantation Immunology," *Journal of the American Medical Association* 258(20):2993-99, November 1987.

Rieger, P. "Immunology: Monoclonal Antibodies," *American Journal of Nursing* 87(4):469-73, April 1987.

Smith, S. "Immunosuppressive Drugs Used in Clinical Practice," *Critical Care Quarterly* 9(1):19-24, June 1986.

White, K. "Treating Pediatric AIDS and Special Precautions for Managing Pediatric AIDS," *AIDS Patient Care* 5-8, 10-12, September 1987.

Index

i refers to an illustration; t refers to a table

Index

i refers to an illustration; t refers to a table

Index

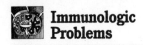

i refers to an illustration; t refers to a table